"The Unobtrusive Relational Analyst *draws on the history of psychoanalysis so as to create its bright future. In its pages the contributions of Freud and British Object Relations theory open to the Relational Turn and to a model of 21st century practice that is integrative and innovative. Through multiple, extended vignettes Grossmark illustrates his clinical position of gentle presence with a remarkable openness and clarity, emphasizing the role of action in the talking cure and the importance of engagement in a process that takes patient and analyst, and will also take the reader, to undiscovered areas of psychic life and living. If this sounds different and new to you, you're right, it is! Transcending parochial divisions, Grossmark creates from varied facets of analytic theory an elegant and eloquent original synthesis that is at once 'in the tradition' and its forward edge.*"

—**Bruce Reis, Ph.D.**, NYU Postdoctoral Program
in Psychotherapy and Psychoanalysis, & the Institute
for Psychoanalytic Training and Research

"*In this wonderfully innovative book, Robert Grossmark shows us how to work with the most difficult patients we encounter, those whose words are empty, whose feelings are dead and who are unable to relate as whole objects or to make a life they can own. Calling on a wide variety of theories from many different schools of thought, Grossmark has woven a conceptual net that captures his unique way of 'companioning' these people whom he describes in such loving and dramatic detail. A companion is someone who travels along with you and shares your bread. I can think of no better companion for a deep psychoanalytic voyage than Robert Grossmark. This book should be a must read for anyone who works with these challenging patients.*"

—**Sheldon Bach, Ph.D.**, Adjunct Clinical Professor of
Psychology, New York University Postdoctoral
Program in Psychoanalysis; Fellow, International
Psychoanalytical Association

The Unobtrusive Relational Analyst

Psychoanalysts increasingly find themselves working with patients and states that are not amenable to verbal and dialogic engagement. Such patients are challenging for a psychoanalytic approach that assumes that the patient relates in the verbal realm and is capable of reflective function. Both the classical stance of neutrality and abstinence and a contemporary relational approach that works with mutuality and intersubjectivity can often ask too much of patients.

The Unobtrusive Relational Analyst introduces a new psychoanalytic register for working with such patients and states, involving a present and engaged analyst who is unobtrusive to the unfolding of the patient's inner world and the flow of mutual enactments. For the unobtrusive relational analyst, the world and idiom of the patient becomes the defining signature of the clinical interaction and process. Rather than seeking to bring patients into greater dialogic relatedness, the analyst companions the patient in the flow of enactive engagement and into the damaged and constrained landscapes of their inner worlds. Being known and companioned in these areas of deep pain, shame and fragmentation is the foundation on which psychoanalytic transformation and healing rests.

In a series of illuminating chapters that include vivid examples drawn from his work with individuals and with groups, Robert Grossmark illustrates the work of the unobtrusive relational analyst. He reconfigures the role of action and enactment in psychoanalysis and group analysis, and expands the understanding of the analyst's subjectivity to embrace receptivity, surrender and companioning. Offering fresh concepts regarding therapeutic action and psychoanalytic engagement, *The Unobtrusive Relational Analyst* will be of great interest to all psychoanalysts and psychoanalytic psychotherapists.

Robert Grossmark is a psychoanalyst working with individuals, couples and groups in New York City. He is Adjunct Clinical Professor and Consultant at the New York University Postdoctoral Program in Psychoanalysis and Psychotherapy. He teaches at the National Institute for the Psychotherapies; the Clinical Psychology Doctoral Program at the City College of New York and the Eastern Group Psychotherapy Society.

The Unobtrusive Relational Analyst

Explorations in Psychoanalytic Companioning

Robert Grossmark

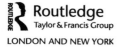
Routledge
Taylor & Francis Group

LONDON AND NEW YORK

First published 2018
by Routledge
2 Park Square, Milton Park, Abingdon, Oxon OX14 4RN

and by Routledge
711 Third Avenue, New York, NY 10017

Routledge is an imprint of the Taylor & Francis Group, an informa business

British Library Cataloguing-in-Publication Data
A catalogue record for this book is available from the British Library

Library of Congress Cataloging-in-Publication Data
Names: Grossmark, Robert, author.
Title: The unobtrusive relational analyst : explorations in psychoanalytic companioning / Robert Grossmark.
Description: Abingdon, Oxon ; New York, NY : Routledge, 2018. | Series: Relational perspectives book series ; v. 101 | Includes bibliographical references and index.
Identifiers: LCCN 2017056381 (print) | LCCN 2017057233 (ebook) | ISBN 9781315708096 (Master) | ISBN 9781317481829 (Web PDF) | ISBN 9781317481812 (ePub) | ISBN 9781317481805 (Mobipocket/Kindle) | ISBN 9781138899056 (hbk. : alk. paper) | ISBN 9781138899063 (pbk. : alk. paper) | ISBN 9781315708096 (ebk)
Subjects: | MESH: Psychoanalytic Therapy | Psychotherapeutic Processes | Professional-Patient Relations | Empathy | Trust
Classification: LCC RC480.5 (ebook) | LCC RC480.5 (print) | NLM WM 460.6 | DDC 616.89/14—dc23
LC record available at https://lccn.loc.gov/2017056381

ISBN: 978-1-138-89905-6 (hbk)
ISBN: 978-1-138-89906-3 (pbk)
ISBN: 978-1-315-70809-6 (ebk)

Typeset in Times New Roman
by Apex CoVantage, LLC

For Carina, Tomas and Sophia

Contents

Prologue

It has always seemed to me that there is something potentially transformational and healing in much human interaction. Life can be a series of confirmations that only support and consolidate what we already believe and anticipate, or life can offer new, unanticipated and even surprising experiences. All of our lives involve some blend of both of these tendencies, but our engagements with others are never neutral. There is never nothing happening between two or more people – neurologically, psychophysiologically, or psychologically. Something is always going on. It could be said that the work of psychoanalysis is to harness that something that always goes on when people engage with each other in the service of healing and transformation.

I state this in broad terms because my experiences have taught me that mutual human impact and transformation evolve in many ways, some obscure and subtle, others quite obvious. Sometimes we engage in verbal interaction, persuasion, and influence. We ask for trust and for a listening ear as we make suggestions and offer our thoughts, opinions, or interpretations. We hope for a listening and receptive mind that will understand and receive what we say with the very meaning we intend. We offer our selves to others and respond to each other with our bodies and minds. If we allow it, we change and grow. From my earliest years in the field of clinical psychology, I have been aware of the many dimensions and forms that change and healing can take.

I began my clinical training as a young man in the United Kingdom (UK) in the early 1980s. At that time, there were only a handful of Clinical Psychology graduate programs in the UK. The field had yet to develop into the burgeoning and popular area of study that is the case today, and all of the programs were predominantly behavioral in orientation. I attended a highly regarded program at the University of Birmingham whose major theoretical orientation was radical Skinnerian behaviorism. Hence we were taught those behavior modification interventions that many of you will recall from your undergraduate courses in psychology: implosion, systematic-desensitization, flooding, and so forth. Treatments were brief, and the professors espoused grave skepticism regarding a relatively new book, Donald Meichenbaum's *Cognitive Behavioral Modification* (1977) because it engaged with the black box of the mind. They were exclusively interested in observable and measurable behavior and regarded Meichenbaum's interest in cognitive process as virtually heretical. Psychoanalysis was regarded as no more developed than witchcraft. You will not be surprised to learn that I found this program stultifying and much of the clinical teaching to be empty of anything that even at that young age I regarded as human.

I did, however, have much involvement with many patients at various externships and clinical placements that took me to inpatient wards in old Victorian Psychiatric Hospitals, outpatient centers in underserved inner city neighborhoods, and National Health clinics. Along with my colleagues, we would conduct the latest and supposedly most effective behavioral interventions. At times, I must say I felt more like I was participating in a surreal Monty Python sketch rather than an endeavor of human healing and care. I do recall standing on the roof of a very high building on the University of Birmingham campus with Barry, a man suffering from a fear of heights. We were doing "flooding"! The wind was howling, and I could barely hang on to my jacket let alone my neat professional clip-pad onto which were clamped the leaves of the SUDS scale. For those of you not schooled in this pseudo-technology, this stands for the Subjective Units of Distress Scale developed in 1969 by Joseph Wolpe (1969) by which one can measure by the subject's report exactly how much distress he or she is experiencing. The gale swept around us, and we could barely hear each other's words. I recall yelling "On a scale of 1 to 10, how would you rate your distress at this moment?" I could barely make out the poor fellow's response. "What did you say?" he screamed into the gale as he clung to the sides of the protruding chimney.

My point is not simply to share with you one of many surreal and zany moments of my early training but to recount that when Barry and I finally took the elevator down to earth's level and walked across the quad to the psychology department, he began to talk about his relationship with his father. His eyes filled with tears and, walking side by side in slightly less gale-force wind on ground level, I too was filled with emotion. We stopped, looked at each other, and proceeded to talk about his family, his father, and the terrible sense of guilt and remorse in his life. And you know what? He began over the next few weeks to feel helped. His fears abated. We continued with the zany behavioral protocol, but it was our talking, our connection, that, even at that age, I was quite clear was the source of his healing and change. Of course, statistically speaking, his was another phobic case treated successfully by behavioral intervention. Barry and I knew otherwise.

I found my way to the few clinical placements that were psychoanalytically oriented and found the handful of psychoanalytic supervisors in Birmingham who had been trained at either the Tavistock or the Hampstead Clinic. I began to breathe easier and dove deep into psychoanalytic texts and theory. As I entered the last few months of the training program, I was bewildered that almost all my classmates in the program believed that they were equipped to be clinical psychologists. I felt that I had barely scratched the surface and was determined to explore further the riches I was beginning to unearth. In the University of Birmingham library, I found a book called *Psychoanalysis and Behavioral Therapy* by Paul Wachtel (1977) and was fascinated by its integrative and respectful tone. Sensing that I had found a bridge from one world to another, I wrote to the author and before long was wending my way across the Atlantic to interview for a place in the Clinical Psychology doctoral program at the City University of New York with Paul Wachtel. I was fortunate enough to be accepted and the rest, as they say, is history.

Along with the delights and challenges of living in New York City, the City University doctoral program offered a unique opportunity to become immersed in the riches of psychoanalytic theory: Freud, Klein, Winnicott, Bion, Kohut, Jacobson, and many others formed the coordinates of a psychoanalytic vision along with meticulous attention to moment-to-moment clinical process. I had found a psychoanalytic home. Those years of learning have been a reliable and fertile ground on which I still plant my psychoanalytic feet, and I still favor careful study of the details of clinical process when engaged in my own psychoanalytic work and that of my supervisees. That initial flourishing of almost wondrous discovery was deepened and filled out some years later during my psychoanalytic training at the New York University Postdoctoral Program in Psychoanalysis and Psychotherapy, where I now supervise and teach. The multi-track system of the program enables a candidate to sample classes and in-depth supervision from many different perspectives and captures an idyll of psychoanalytic multiplicity and cosmopolitanism.[1] At "Postdoc," every theory offers something unique, and theories and perspectives engage in ongoing mutual, respectful, and transformative dialogue. Something larger than the sum of the parts emerges and generates its own lively and vibrant psychoanalysis, which feels to me to be more relevant than ever in today's world where subjectivity and truth are under daily assault.

The psychoanalysis that I now reside within is a vibrant contemporary enterprise. The relational turn foregrounded the intersubjective and mutual aspects of the relationship and reconfigured the analytic situation to a more egalitarian and participatory endeavor, a shift that so many have found more welcoming and approachable. However, it seems to me that more and more we are met with patients who are unable to engage with these aspects of a contemporary psychoanalytic treatment. We find many patients who, as a result of early trauma and neglect, do not experience themselves in their own subjectivity and live in very different and unique inner realities. They might not recognize the other as a separate and coherent individual and cannot express their inner struggles and confusion in words or organized thoughts. Whether this is the gradual emergence of a new category of psychological emptiness and confusion emanating from the demands of our contemporary existence is a question for research and debate. In my clinical experience over a number of decades working in inpatient psychiatric units, various outpatient mental health clinics, and in my private practice, I have struggled with the challenge that such patients and states offer to psychoanalytic practice.

The challenge that I take up in this book is how to preserve and find the potential healing qualities of the human encounter in the psychoanalytic situation with patients for whom the human encounter itself is deeply constrained and other. How do we work psychoanalytically with patients and states that are not available for verbal, cognitively organized engagement and relatedness? How can we be present as ourselves and not rely on – or some might say, hide behind – a mystique of neutrality and abstinence while allowing the patient's world, idiom, and true self to grow and fill the treatment? How do we offer ourselves to the other for use and growth and respect the primacy of the patient's inner reality, however opaque and divergent it may be? How do we respect and engage with the patient's lived, conscious experience and value and welcome the full expression of the patient's unconscious life? I hope that my ideas on the unobtrusive relational analyst, the flow of enactive engagement, psychoanalytic companioning, and the eloquence of action described in the following pages will offer some answers or at least spirited engagements with these questions.

Note

1 I borrow the phrase "cosmopolitanism" from Kwame Anthony Appiah (2006), whose work on integrating multiple identities and cultures has influenced and moved me.

References

Appiah, K. W. (2006). *Cosmopolitanism: Ethics in a world of strangers*. New York: Norton.

Meichenbaum, D. (1977). *Cognitive behavior modification: An integrative approach*. New York: Plenum Press.

Wachtel, P. (1977). *Psychoanalysis and behavior therapy: Toward an integration*. New York: Basic Books.

Wolpe, J. (1969). *The practice of behavioral therapy*. New York: Pergamon Press.

Acknowledgements

First and foremost, I must express my deep gratitude to all of my patients who have allowed me into their inner worlds over the past 40 years. Each treatment is a journey, and I have had so many brave, resilient, and creative fellow travelers. Each and every one has taught me something new.

I have had the good fortune to teach and supervise in a number of institutes and programs over the years. I would like to thank all my students and supervisees at the New York University Postdoctoral Program in Psychotherapy and Psychoanalysis, the doctoral program in clinical psychology at City College of New York, The National Institute for the Psychotherapies, The Eastern Group Psychotherapy Society, and the Minnesota Institute for Contemporary Psychotherapy and Psychoanalysis. You have all nourished and challenged me. You have inspired me to develop my thoughts and to spell them out as clearly as possible.

I also thank all those who attend my reading and teaching groups. The commitment to serious learning, good humor, and camaraderie is quite wonderful and never fails to energize and uplift. I thank you for allowing me the opportunity to share and develop my clinical perspective with you.

I want to acknowledge and thank all those who have helped me with this volume. In particular, I want to thank Shelly Bach, Donnel Stern, Bruce Reis, and Carina Grossmark, who read drafts of the chapters that comprise this book and gave helpful feedback, guidance, and support.

I have attended a reading group led by Donnel Stern for many years. This unique learning environment has been invaluable for the development of my own clinical voice, and I especially want to thank Don and all the other members of the group: Lisa Director, Orna Guralnik, Arthur Heiserman, Katherine Leddick, James Ogilvie, Deborah Rothschild, and Liz Weiss.

I have so many wonderful colleagues and professional friends and cannot hope to make mention of every single one here. However, I do want to express my gratitude to a number of colleagues who consciously and unconsciously have helped shape my thinking and have inspired me to grow and write: Bruce Reis, Lisa Director, Asher Kahn, Jama Adams, Fred Stern, Steven Tublin, Philip Blumberg; in London Keith Miller; in Tel Aviv, Michal Rieck, Meir and Smadar Steinbock, and in Jerusalem, Shlomit Haber-Mosheiov. Among the many wonderful supervisors from whom I learned over the years I especially want to thank Philip Bromberg, Doris Silverman, Jim Fosshage, and Ronnie Levine. I owe a special debt of gratitude to Shelly Bach for many years of transformational supervision and guidance.

I wish to thank my dear friends Howard Levi and Alexandra Avlonitis and Asher Kahn and Sheri Katz for many years of friendship and support, and I thank Alexandra for permission to use her beautiful painting for the cover of this volume.

I thank Kristopher Spring for diligent editing and helpful guidance, and many thanks to Kate Hawes and Charles Bath at Routledge for support and help in bringing this volume to print.

Many thanks and gratitude to Lew Aron and Adrienne Harris for inviting me to contribute this volume to the Relational Perspectives book series. It is a great pleasure and an honor to be a part of this book series that has transformed the way we think about and practice psychoanalysis.

Finally, there are no words to express my gratitude to my wife, Carina Grossmark, who has not only supported me in my life, my professional development, and writing but has really been instrumental in making it happen at all. Despite the demands of her own busy schedule, she read every word of this book and has consistently been my most perceptive and creative editor.

I express my thanks to all the journals and publishers who have granted permission for me to reprint articles and quotations in this volume.

Chapter 1, The Unobtrusive Relational Analyst was originally published in *Psychoanalytic Dialogues*, (2012), 22:629–646. Reprinted with kind permission by Taylor & Francis, LLC.

The epigraphs in Chapter 1 by Hans Loewald and in Chapter 6 by Oz and Oz-Salzberger are reprinted with the kind permission of Yale University Press.

Chapter 2, The Flow of Enactive Engagement was originally published in *Contemporary Psychoanalysis*, (2012) 48, 3, 287–300. Reprinted with kind permission of Taylor & Francis, LLC.

The Matthew Sanford epigraph featured at the start of Chapter 3 is reprinted by kind permission of Rodale, Inc.

Chapter 3, Psychoanalytic Companioning was originally published in *Psychoanalytic Dialogues*, (2016) 26: 698–712. Reprinted with kind permission of Taylor & Francis, LLC.

The epigraph quotation from Paul Williams in Chapter 4 is also reprinted with kind permission of Taylor & Francis, LLC.

The epigraph in Chapter 5 by John Ashbery is reprinted with the kind permission of Georges Bourchardt, Inc.

The epigraph in Chapter 6 by Tomas Trastromer is reprinted with the kind permission of Harper Collins.

The first epigraph featured in Chapter 7 by H. Porter Abbot is reprinted with the kind permission of the Cambridge University Press.

The second epigraph featured in Chapter 7 is an excerpt from "The Uses of Story" from *Making Stories* by Jerome Bruner. Copyright © 2002 by Jerome Bruner. Reprinted by permission of Farrar, Straus and Giroux.

The epigraph featured in Chapter 8 by Bela Bartok is an excerpt from *Bela Bartok: Letters* edited by J. Demeny and is reprinted with the kind permission of Faber & Faber.

Sections of Chapter 7 appeared in Robert Grossmark's "The Case of Pamela" originally published in *Psychoanalytic Dialogues* (2009), Vol. 19, 1, 22–30. Reprinted with the kind permission of Taylor & Francis, LLC.

Sections of Chapter 7 also appeared in Robert Grossmark's "Two Men Talking: The Emergence of Multiple Masculinities in Psychoanalytic Treatment" originally published in B. Reis and R. Grossmark (Eds) *Heterosexual Masculinities: Contemporary Perspectives from Psychoanalytic Gender Theory*. Co-editor. New York: Routledge, Taylor & Francis Group (2009). Reprinted with the kind permission of Taylor & Francis, LLC.

Sections of Chapter 9 were originally published in Robert Grossmark's "Narrating the Unsayable: Enactment, Repair and Creative Multiplicity in Group Psychotherapy" originally published in the *International Journal of Group Psychotherapy*, (2017) Vol. 67, 1: 27–46. Reprinted with the kind permission of Taylor & Francis, LLC.

Sections of Chapter 10 were originally published in Robert Grossmark's "The Unobtrusive Relational Group Psychotherapist and the Work of the Narrative" to be published in *Psychoanalytic Inquiry*, Spring 2018. Reprinted with the kind permission of Taylor & Francis, LLC.

Introduction

> We must be prepared to assume the existence in us of not only a second consciousness, but of a third, fourth, perhaps of an unlimited number of states of consciousness, all unknown to us and to one another.
> —Sigmund Freud (1915, p. 170)

States of consciousness that do not take the form of verbal and cognizable mental contents have always presented a challenge for psychoanalytic treatment and for mental health treatment in general. Freud's great opus primarily addressed the repressed unconscious that lent itself to psychodynamic formulations, oedipal conflict, and the treatment of the neuroses. But as his comment quoted above and his delineation of the unrepressed unconscious suggest (Freud, 1923),[1] there are many more levels and dimensions to conscious and non-conscious life and experience. Many of these dimensions do not take the form of organized thoughts or cognitions and are not bound by the structures afforded by verbal language. Such areas typically become known via sensation, diffuse bodily experience, action and motility, dreams and hallucinatory phenomena, overwhelming anxiety states, and via what we now term enactment.

Psychoanalytic treatment has tended to struggle with these areas of the human and has generally tilted to creating form where there was diffusion, language where there was merely sound, thoughts where there was raw sensation, and consciousness where there was the unconscious. Often, psychoanalytic treatment eschewed patients who did not rely primarily on language and consequently could not engage with both the structure and the spirit of the psychoanalytic endeavor, seeing them as too narcissistic, disorganized, or primitive. Action, motility, and pure sensation tended to be classed as acting out, resistances, or assaults on the treatment.

In recent years, there has been a resurgence of interest in mental states and processes that lie outside of the organized and cognized dynamic unconscious. From the relational/interpersonal psychoanalytic world, Donnel Stern's (1997, 2010, 2015) ground-breaking work on unformulated experience exercises a large influence here, as does Christopher Bollas's (1987) conception of the unthought known, the work of Levine et al. (2013) on unrepresented states, Andre Green's (1999) work on the negative, Sheldon Bach's (1985, 2006, 2016) embrace of altered states of consciousness and existence, and many more.

The relational turn ushered in a new era of psychoanalysis. We now comfortably regard psychoanalytic process as a mutual and egalitarian endeavor. While this mutuality is not symmetrical (Aron, 1996), the contemporary relational psychoanalyst now uses expressions of his or her own subjectivity with a freedom and creativity and is not silenced by the arbitrary constraints of "abstinence" and "neutrality." No longer regarded as situated on a perch outside of the interaction (D. B. Stern, 1997) with a "view from nowhere" (Nagel, 1986), the contemporary analyst gains insight and fosters the analytic process from a position that allows him or her to be "seen, moved, disrupted and reconfigured" within the treatment process (Wright, 2015, p.27). Moving beyond the view of the human mind as both unitary and sealed, current psychoanalytic process is viewed as hinging on the interaction of the subjectivities of both psychoanalyst and analysand and as embedded in complex social and historical contexts. In addition to the classical psychoanalytic focus on transference and its resolution as the fulcrum of the psychoanalytic cure, the relational turn privileged the centrality of enactments that involve both analyst and analysand, and the progress of many relational treatments often hinges on the emergence and resolution of these enactments. Overall, Relational theory seems to have picked up a climate change in contemporary psychoanalytic and psychotherapy culture that yearns for more human and egalitarian relatedness between patients and analysts, and a view that sees such relatedness as integral to psychoanalytic cure rather than as a contamination of a scientific process.

While all these transformations have enabled so many of us to breathe more easily as psychoanalysts and work with creativity and engagement, the relational field has also struggled to find ways to work with patients who are constrained – sometimes severely – in their ability to engage in dialogic exploration and who barely experience continuity of the self or subjectivity in themselves or in others, including the analyst. For such patients, interpretations about inner conflict or consideration of the dynamics in the treatment interaction with the analyst are potentially voices from another world. They may comply and utilize their verbal, related selves, but their inner core will remain at best untouched and at worst shamed into disavowal and inner sequestration. I am also referring here to patients who may appear to be more developed and may present with, and be able to engage in, what can appear to be intersubjective vitality. However, many patients who present in this way also harbor self-states that contain earlier undeveloped, empty, unspeakable, and profoundly non-related parts of themselves that can find no expression in language. These areas of the self are much less likely to be reached by dialogic engagement and are often chased underground or shamed by a psychoanalytic treatment that puts a premium on relatedness, thought, and verbal exploration.

This volume engages with these patients and states. The spirit of this volume is the endeavor to be unobtrusive to the incarnation of other states of consciousness and psychological organization as they emerge in the treatment. These are arisings of the non-represented, non-symbolized, and unformulated that announce their presence in alternate registers – motoric, sensory, hallucinatory, oneiric, reverie, and above all, action. Rather than orienting our analytic work to moving the patient out of these regressed areas into greater relatedness, we welcome these other dimensions and their full expression within the analytic sphere in mutual regression and mutual enactment. We orient ourselves to going further *in* to these emerging worlds of confusion, trauma, and pain rather than seeking to peremptorily draw the patient *out* of these areas. Such regressions and emergences in the analytic field are understood as silent screams from within the patient, who is crying out to be joined with and known in these inner worlds of torment and suffering, rather than pulled out of them and thus potentially shamed and abandoned. The treatment belongs to the patient, and it is the analyst's work to find and join with the register and wavelength that is the truest expression of the patient's inner world and experience. From this perspective, enactments are regarded as transpersonal narrations of what is beyond language and symbolization. They emerge as inscriptions on the field of the treatment and involve both participants (or all participants in group analysis) and often defy neat and organized verbal understanding and description. Hence psychoanalytic healing and psychological growth and differentiation take hold when the psychoanalyst can unobtrusively companion the patient into areas of non-developed, non-related, and non-represented inner life in the register that is organic to the patient at that time. In so doing, the unrepresented and unformulated take spontaneous form and are embellished in enactment between the analytic partners and in the field.

From this point of view, our understanding of our patients and clinical process takes into account both the ongoing and ineluctable intersubjective nature of the subject *and* honors and welcomes the private and secluded areas of the patient's conscious and unconscious inner worlds. This embraces the paradoxes at the center of Winnicott's (1958) rendition of the human condition: We are all embedded in our environments *and* we are all essentially isolates; the capacity to be alone is central to our ability to connect to others with vitality and authenticity.

In this book, I spell out a psychoanalytic register that seeks to work with these patients and states in their own idiom and form. In so doing, I have sought to square the circle of allowing – and welcoming – the patient to be free to manifest all the dimensions of their being – however diffuse and confused – unencumbered by the requirements of relatedness *and* for the analyst to be real and present while tilting their subjectivity to be receptive to the developmental and present needs of the patient. This is the work of the unobtrusive relational analyst.

Organization of this book

The book is organized into two separate parts. The first part, "Psychoanalytic process," addresses the clinical theory and approach of the unobtrusive relational analyst and deals with psychoanalytic work with individual analysands. Each chapter addresses different vectors of unobtrusive relational psychoanalytic work and introduces various phenomena that arise and come to reside in the analytic space when the analyst is unobtrusive to their full expression.

The second part, "Group analysis," addresses my work with groups. I offer extensive examples from my group work that broaden the reach and deepen the feel for the approach of the unobtrusive relational analyst.

Chapter 1, "The unobtrusive relational analyst," addresses the challenge of working as a relational psychoanalyst with non-alive and non-speakable states and ways of being. The chapter builds upon the contemporary relational sensibility that values the intersubjective engagement of analyst and patient and the enactment of dissociated and unformulated states and integrates the concepts of regression and the unobtrusive analyst that were central to the work of Michael and Enid Balint and the British Independent group. I outline the approach of the unobtrusive relational analyst, who is neither neutral nor abstinent and is both deeply engaged with the patient and simultaneously surrenders to the developmental and archaic needs of the patient to be the analyst the patient needs him to be. This can often involve tolerating experiences and sessions that seem far from what we might otherwise regard as psychoanalysis. I describe my work with a patient that was enhanced and made possible by my engaged but unobtrusive presence and the privileging of the patient's own idiom, object relating, and early developmental needs. This chapter emphasizes that far from withholding the analyst's subjectivity, the unobtrusive relational analyst engages deeply with the patient's inner world and creates an impactful analytic intimacy. This is a theme that is carried in every chapter of this book, and it is this depth of engagement that is at core to the healing that I describe in each of the chapters.

In Chapter 2, I offer a concept of therapeutic action that I call "The Flow of Enactive Engagement" that is the fulcrum of a contemporary psychoanalytic treatment, just as free association was once to classical psychoanalysis. The analyst and analysand live within the field of the treatment that is created by the two participants but is greater than the sum of its parts. Just as Freud (1913) saw free association as the road to psychoanalytic cure and advised the analyst to not intrude on the analysand's associations, I suggest that an unobtrusive relational analyst can allow the process of the field to emerge and tell its own story. This approach is distinguished from the traditional interpersonal/relational approach that foregrounds examination of the therapeutic interaction as the key to therapeutic action.

Chapter 3 delineates the concept of "Psychoanalytic Companioning." When working with patients and states where there is no self-other definition and therefore no mutuality, the path to healing and growth is via companioning the patient into the darker, more regressed, and unformed states of illusion and merger rather than via the promotion of separateness and relatedness, which, I suggest, arise spontaneously and with the imprint of the patient's authentic self within the companioned register of the analysis. This chapter emphasizes that it is going *with* the patient into his or her inner world of pain and turmoil that is healing rather than attempts to pull the patient out of their own register into a more organized and conventionally related dimension. This involves a different register of the analyst's subjectivity: one that is receptive, "cooperative" (Trevarthen, 2001), and responsive to the patient's internal world and objects rather than analytic and knowing.

Chapter 4, "The eloquence of action: unobtrusive psychoanalytic companioning and the growth of mind and self," summarizes the concepts outlined in the first three chapters and foregrounds the value of welcoming the expression of the patient's inchoate and non-symbolized states and ways of being into the treatment. The focus is on mutual action and motoric and sensorial communication. I argue for an understanding of somatic and motoric impulsion as a dimension of mentalization rather than as counter-therapeutic "acting out." Such behavioral emanations in the treatment are not regarded as *not* thinking, but are welcomed as thinking *in another register*. This is the eloquence of action.

In Chapter 5, "Enactment: the total situation," I take up Klein's concept of total situations and Betty Joseph's (1985) subsequent elaboration of transference as a total situation. Some treatments involve a regression to a total situation, a monolithic and totalistic experience of every aspect of the analytic treatment that becomes incarnated in the flow of enactive engagement and involves both analyst and patient. Often, the analyst will feel annulled and hopeless in the face of a total situation. When the analyst is unobtrusive to the emergence of these total situations and resides within them together with the patient, other states and possibilities emerge spontaneously and can free the patient from the deathly grip of early toxic identifications.

In total situations and other regressions to altered dimensions of being, the experience of time and space is suspended or altered. Chapter 6, "Everything happens at once: the emergence of symmetric enactment," addresses the timeless and spaceless dimension of the unrepressed unconscious. The unobtrusive relational analyst can expect to live within altered states with patients whose orientation to reality, time, and space are undeveloped or suffused with the sediments of inconsistent and sometimes bizarre early objects and trauma. I develop the concept of "symmetric enactment," which captures the mutual enactment of timelessness and spacelessness, and offer a vignette that tells of how I came to companion one patient in a zone with no time, space, and differentiation.

A thread that runs through all the chapters in this book is the idea that enactments tell a story. Enactments are conceptualized as narrations and representations in action of what has yet to assume a form. In Chapter 7, "The work of the narrative and enactive co-narration," I develop the concept of enactive co-narration. Building on Bollas's (2009) idea that there is a human drive to represent, I suggest that when the analyst can be unobtrusive to the flourishing of the authentic idiom of the patient, trauma and the unknown self come to take representational shape and form in the flow of enactive engagement in the mutually constructed field.

The second part of this volume addresses the application of the principles and theory thus far outlined to work as a group analyst. Groups contain the potential for creativity, growth, and healing as well as hate and destructiveness that reside whenever humans come together. The psychoanalytic group literature has, I believe, tended to emphasize the regressive and destructive aspects of group interaction, emphasizing the resistant quality of early, primitive defenses and dynamics in group functioning as well as promoting the role of group leader or therapist as neutral, abstinent, and above the fray. In these chapters, I outline a vision of psychoanalytic group work where what has been regarded as destructive and resistant phenomena are construed as enactments that capture untold and untellable narratives of trauma and pain. Rather than simply destructive, I take such phenomena as having creative potential. I see the group analyst as both sharing the group experience as it unfolds as well as functioning as a container for these sometimes turbulent experiences. The group analyst does not function as the one who knows but lends his or her reflective function to the group such that the members can make their own meaning and their own stories. The analyst is unobtrusive to the development of each group's own idiom and character.

In this volume, enactment is regarded as an ongoing and ubiquitous process. Chapter 8, "The edge of chaos: enactment, disruption, and emergence in group psychotherapy," lays out the idea that groups are inevitably and constantly shifting in and out of enactments and that there is a constant dialectic between thinking and not thinking, relating and not relating in group process. This chapter looks to nonlinear dynamic systems theory – or chaos theory – to explicate this process. The chapter emphasizes a core principle of this kind of group work: that the treatment is by the group. The group analyst is regarded as embedded within the unfolding enactments rather than outside of them, and the leader's role is to shepherd this process and to support the group in developing its own character, language, and healing as it engages in the creative hermeneutic work of making meaning out of chaos.

Chapter 9, "Narrating the unsayable: enactment, repair, and creative multiplicity in group psychotherapy," introduces the core relational concepts of dissociation, enactment, and unformulated experience and applies them to working with groups. The application of these concepts to the work of the group-as-a-whole and clinical examples of the emergence of powerful enactments of trauma and internalized deadness offer a window into this challenging and vibrant work.

Chapter 10, "The unobtrusive relational group analyst and the work of the narrative," outlines a vision of group treatment where the group enters the flow of enactive engagement with the leader and the other group members such that members companion each other into the darker and more regressed, non-symbolized areas of their individual minds and of the group mind. The emphasis is on the emergence of narratives between the group members and between the group and the leader that hitherto had no form or representation.

The major thrust of this volume is to find ways to work with and join patients and groups in their own idiom, register, and states of consciousness so that they can fill out and own their own treatment and thus their own selves and lives. The unobtrusive relational analyst offers a different dimension of the analyst's subjectivity and is present as him- or herself while surrendering to analysands' inchoate striving to represent themselves in the unique organism that emerges in each particular psychoanalytic pair. The emphasis is on the quality of with-ness that grows in the treatment. This approach gives full due to the psychoanalytic primacy of what is not conscious and is yet to be formulated, known, or symbolized. To return to the epigraph of this introduction, this work offers an embrace of "not only a second consciousness, but of a third, fourth, perhaps of an unlimited number of states of consciousness" (Freud, 1915, p. 170), and it is our work as analysts to discover and create these with our patients.

Note

1 In "The Ego and The Id," Freud (1923) writes: "We recognize that the Unc. does not coincide with the repressed; it is still true that all that is repressed is

Ucs. But not all that is Ucs. is repressed. A part of the ego, too – and Heaven knows how important a part – may be Ucs., undoubtedly is Ucs." (p. 18).

References

Aron, L. (1996). *A meeting of minds: Mutuality in psychoanalysis*. Hillsdale, NJ: The Analytic Press.

Bach, S. (1985). *Narcissistic states and the therapeutic process*. Northvale, NJ: Jason Aronson.

Bach, S. (2006). *Getting from here to there: Analytic love, analytic process*. Hillsdale, NJ: The Analytic Press.

Bach, S. (2016). *Chimeras and other writings: Selected papers of Sheldon Bach*. Astoria, NY: International Psychoanalytic Books.

Bollas, C. (1987). *The shadow of the object: Psychoanalysis of the unthought known*. New York: Columbia University Press.

Bollas, C. (2009). Free association. In C. Bollas, *The evocative object world* (pp. 5–46). London: Routledge.

Freud, S. (1913). Further recommendations on the technique of psychoanalysis: On beginning the treatment. In J. Strachey (Ed. & Trans.), *The standard edition of the complete psychological works of Sigmund Freud* (Vol. 12, pp. 121–144). London: Hogarth Press.

Freud, S. (1915). The unconscious. In J. Strachey (Ed. & Trans.), *The standard edition of the complete psychological works of Sigmund Freud* (Vol. 14, pp. 19–213). London: Hogarth Press.

Freud, S. (1923). The ego and the id. In J. Strachey (Ed. & Trans.), *The standard edition of the complete psychological works of Sigmund Freud* (Vol. 19, pp. 1–66). London: Hogarth Press.

Green, A. (1999). *The work of the negative*. London: Free Association Books.

Joseph, B. (1985). Transference: The total situation. In M. Feldman & E. B. Spillius (Eds.), *Psychic equilibrium and psychic change: Selected papers of Betty Joseph* (pp. 156–167). London: Routledge.

Levine, H., Reed, G. S., & Scarfone, D. (Eds.). (2013). *Unrepresented states and the construction of meaning: Clinical and theoretical contributions*. London: Karnac Books.

Nagel, T. (1986). *The view from nowhere*. New York: Oxford University Press.

Stern, D. B. (1997). *Unformulated experience: From dissociation to imagination in psychoanalysis*. Hillsdale, NJ: The Analytic Press.

Stern, D. B. (2010). *Partners in thought: Working with unformulated experience, dissociation and enactment*. New York: Routledge.

Stern, D. B. (2015). *Relational freedom: Emergent properties of the relational field*. London: Routledge.

Trevarthen, C. (2001). Intrinsic motives for companionship in understanding: Their origin, development, and the significance for infant mental health. *Infant Mental Health Journal, 22*(1–2), 95–131.

Winnicott, D. W. (1958). The capacity to be alone. In D. W. Winnicott, *The maturational processes and the facilitating environment* (pp. 29–36). New York: International Universities Press.

Wright, F. (2015). Being seen, moved, disrupted and reconfigured: Group leadership from a relational perspective. In R. Grossmark & F. Wright (Eds.), *The one and the many: Relational approaches to group psychotherapy* (pp. 27–37). London: Routledge.

Part I

Psychoanalytic process

Chapter 1

The unobtrusive
relational analyst[1]

> *To put it quite pointedly, life itself, and especially individual life and*
> *separateness, are not taken for granted.*
> —Hans Loewald, 'The Waning of the Oedipus Conflict*
> *(Loewald, 1980, p. 399)*

Introduction

I think it's fair to say that from a relational perspective, clinical narrative takes its shape from the intertwining of the subjectivities, and conscious and unconscious processes of both patient and analyst. While some emphasize the role of dissociation and enactment and others have foregrounded the intersubjective matrix of the therapy dyad and the role of implicit relational knowing, I believe there is a common emphasis on careful communication of the analyst's experience or countertransference in the moment as part of the co-creation of the clinical narrative – a version of what Edgar Levenson (1983) has described as a constant orientation to wonder and ask "what's going on around here?" – together with an invitation to the patient to think about and to engage with the analyst's process, conscious or unconscious (Aron, 1996; Bass, 2009). In this more egalitarian and co-participant approach, mutual interaction and influence is privileged. I think that for many contemporary analysts, from many theoretical perspectives, and I dare say, for many patients too, the idea of psychoanalysis as a mutual enterprise has been freeing, inviting, and basically more comfortable and respectful, and in keeping with our current feel for authority relations.

I would like to propose here that addressing the patient-analyst inter-action in the here-and-now is not the *only* way that a relational analyst works, nor is it the way that a treatment with a relational analyst *need* unfold. My suggestion here is that there are other aspects of contemporary relational treatment that reach and allow for the emergence of different registers of the patient's experiences. These, I believe, are less frequently foregrounded in the description of relational psychoanalytic treatment. I will describe a treatment approach that emphasizes an unobtrusive and companioning analytic engagement and illustrate this with a description of a case. I will offer a conceptualization of therapeutic action that embel-lishes and re-casts the psychoanalytic concepts of regression, intersubjec-tivity, and clinical intimacy.

In the effort to describe the clinical phenomena I will be focusing on, I will borrow from various threads of the contemporary psychoanalytic tapestry, including relational, object relations, contemporary Freudian, British independent, self psychology, intersubjective, infant research, and more. I recognize that weaving these together can create some inconsist-encies in language and theory, but I have found that it has been organic to me to proceed in this way in my effort to develop a functional language to convey these clinical experiences.

Without aliveness, reflection, and recognition

When asked to engage in an exploration of mutual influence and "what's-going-on-around-here?" the patient is asked to do collaborative mental work, to "relate." This requires a level of psychological development, an ability to symbolize and mentalize, to think about things, a "reflective self-awareness" (Bach, 1994, 2006). Above all, it requires that the patient be *alive* and that the patient experiences him or her self as a whole person in the presence of another whole and separate person, as a subject with subjective experience in the presence of another subject. The idea that experience is mutually constructed may be theoretically true, but it can sometimes be far from the truth of the patient's actual subjective experi-ence of the analyst and of their own needs.

For patients who do not experience themselves as existing in time and space in a continuous and coherent way, and who do not regard other human beings as whole, coherent, and separate beings, as subjects; it is too much to expect mutuality. Such patients' reality often involves confusion as to whether they are alive or dead, and whether the world, other people, and the self actually exist and can be expected to continue to exist. These damaged self-states may co-exist simultaneously with verbally adept, intellectual and related self-states. I would suggest that treating patients who suffer this way as if they are alive and whole, separate beings may re-traumatize them, and an as-if analysis may be co-constructed. The related and expressive analyst, who can hold up his or her own experience for examination as it relates to the interaction in the treatment, can unwittingly shame and silence such patients, and this can compound the dissociation of the most damaged parts of the patient's inner world.

Bromberg (1996, 2006) and D. B. Stern (2004) have suggested that in treatments of patients dominated by a dissociative structure, the engagement with intrapsychic conflict is the sign that the treatment is reaching a successful end, rather than the resolution of conflict being a necessary part of the cure. Similarly, Slochower (1996) notes that "the intersubjective analytic relationship is a hard-won therapeutic achievement, that often does not emerge until well into the treatment process" (p. 33). One might further say that with patients such as those I am talking about, the ability to engage with and recognize an other in the room is the sign that the treatment has worked, rather than the necessary part of the treatment.

The analyst who can analyze his or her own experience and invite the patient to do so may also induce an idealization. In the egalitarian spirit of Ferenczi, relational technique has emphasized the use of ordinary vernacular speech in psychoanalytic treatment. However, it is worth considering that analysts' ability to express and analyze their own experience results in a kind of interaction far from ordinary vernacular conversation, and that kind of interaction, which may be beyond the capacity of the patient, can inadvertently foster deep idealizations. Such an analyst's very humanity can be traumatizing to the parts of the self that are dominated by envy, omnipotence, and shame. I am reminded of Michael Balint's observation that the patients with whom his friend Sandor Ferenczi applied his active and mutual technique showed more, not less, dependency on him (Balint, 1968, p. 174). Ferenczi was working toward an egalitarian relationship; his patients were spellbound by his ability to do this. I think this is sobering and perhaps cautionary.

I am talking here about the analyst's receptivity to patients' experiences of deadness, non-existence, being in bits, or difficulties in simply going on being. The experience of states such as these can be interrupted by an analyst's focus on the verbal realm as expressed, for example, by curiosity and the analyzing of what the patient is doing and/or eliciting in others and in the analyst. Bion talked of the "obtrusive object analyst" as curious, but unable to withstand being the receptacle of parts of the patient's personality that neither patient nor analyst can yet know, much less describe and talk about. (Bion, 1962)

It seems to me that silence, quietness, patience, and not speaking the countertransference have been conflated with "neutrality." Of course, the concepts of "neutrality" and "abstinence" have been deconstructed as reflecting a one-person psychology (Hoffman, 2006). But perhaps an unintentional result of this analysis is that something of Winnicott's paradoxical approach to transitional phenomena has been obscured (Winnicott, 1960). We can accept the relational credo that we continually co-construct experience in analysis, *and* recognize that not all patients *experience* this or are even aware that this might be so, or even that bringing this to the patient's consciousness is always of value. I take from Winnicott (1958) that we are continually situated in the intersubjective matrix *and* that treatment can be allowed to unfold such that areas of psychological being that we are barely able to sense let alone describe in words, can emerge and take shape.

I shall shortly be describing my work with an unusual young man, who overtly rejected any attempts of mine to examine the process between us, and any interpretation of his psychological functioning. He was unusual in that he could clearly ask and even demand a very particular kind of object relationship with me. He was quite clear that he was not alive in the usually accepted use of the term, he did not feel he truly existed, nor did he take as a given that I was a whole person who lived in a coherent chronological and spatial reality. More of him later. My point is that parts of the experience of many patients are damaged in this way. These areas of their minds, or self-states, are rarely described as such by the patients themselves, and can be chased underground by an analyst who may subtly convey that what is needed is a verbal, sentient, related partner/patient to join in relatedness with the analyst, or at least strive to do so. Ogden (1989) talks about the "act of theft" (p. 176) whereby an analyst eager to connect with a patient can rob him or her of the opportunity to inscribe the analysis in the unique way that they consciously and unconsciously choose.

Michael and Enid Balint and the unobtrusive analyst

Writing in the 1960s and basing his thinking on object relations and the Winnicottian-independent-tradition, Michael Balint (1968) describes patients who could not use the standard psychoanalytic technique of the time. Interpretations were of no use to them; he observed that they craved not so much the "gratification of an instinct or drive" (p. 159) as a certain kind of object relationship, one that was "more primitive than that obtaining between two adults" (p. 161). The provision and welcoming of the emergence of that object relationship in the treatment was what could be healing to these patients. I have found his technical recommendations to be very useful and real to me. First and foremost he emphasizes the need "to recognize and be with the patient" (p. 172), and for the analyst to be "unobtrusive and ordinary" (p. 173). In Balint's language, this facilitates a "benign regression" by which Balint means a treatment situation that will promote the emergence of the most "primitive" parts of the patient's functioning, those that are most strongly implicated in the patient's damaged way of being in the world. He distinguishes benign regression from malignant forms of regression that can evolve from the omniscient and omnipotent aspects of the analyst's technique. In Balint's world the omniscient and omnipotent analyst is the one who adheres to and insists on the truth of his or her interpretations. In our contemporary psychoanalytic climate, "omniscience" and "omnipotence" can come in many other forms, including an unexamined tendency to proceed as if discussing the ongoing interaction in the moment is always a good idea – that is, proceeding without considering how working in this way may affect the patient whose facility in this area is not as well developed as the analyst's.

Balint (1968) and his wife Enid Balint (1993), in a sequence of papers on psychoanalytic technique, talk about being "unobtrusive." I read this as distinct from the idea of a neutral or abstinent analyst. Rather, I find much that is useful in the idea of not getting in the way of the relationship that the patient seems to be, and they would say, *needs to* be creating in the treatment. They highlight that the only value from the treatment gained by patients like this – patients with much envy, hatred, and extreme vulnerability – has to be experienced as coming from them, from their minds, their words, and their efforts. This approach need not diverge from the sensibility that experience in the treatment is co-constructed. It does, however, allow the space for these patients to use the co-constructed "field" of treatment in the way that *they* need to, in the moment.

So, how to be with a patient such as this, or with self-states such as this? Balint recognizes the dilemmas involved and speaks of the almost entirely non-verbal medium in phases of a treatment such as this.

> for some years now I have experimented with a technique that allows the patient to experience a two-person relationship which cannot, need not, and perhaps, must not, be expressed in words, but, merely by, 'acting out' in the analytic situation.

(p. 174)

He continues that later, when the patient has emerged from this phase, then the process and the "acting out" can be worked through. Nowadays we might say that when the dissociative structure is recognized, then we can experience and talk about conflict with the patient (Bromberg, 2006; D. B. Stern, 2004). Balint's approach suggests a living through of enactments and waiting for the patient to find the resolution *in their own idiom.* There is concordance here with some contemporary analysts, even as they themselves have differing conceptions of "intersubjectivity." I am thinking of Bruce Reis's recent work on enactive witnessing (Reis, 2009). Reis privileges the silent accompanying and "being-with the patient," as painful traumatic enactments take place in the treatment. A similar angle on the analyst's position is found in much of Christopher Bollas's work, and particularly in his paper on free association (Bollas, 2009). Slochower (1996, 2004) has emphasized that the analyst can utilize a "holding" position when "intersubjective exploration can be disruptive rather than facilitative" (Slochower, 1996, p. 34) With these writers, I do not hear "silence" as the literal silence of "no words," but rather as a tactful and connected "silence," a "with-ness" (Reis, 2011) that does not intrude on the patient's ownership of their own sensations and their own particular experience of the analyst, by knowing more than the patient or even offering the patient more than they create themselves in the moment. We can accompany patients with a "quiet that is not silence" (Reis, 2011) while they "are afloat in the reveries of their own subjectivity" (Bach, 2009, p. 41).

Balint (1968) talks about accepting that for the patient in these times, words are not truly functioning as the means of communication. "They are lifeless, repetitive and stereotyped, they do not mean what they say"

(p. 177). The analyst has to accept this and "abandon any attempt at organizing the material produced by the patient" (p. 177). Accordingly, Balint recommends that "the analyst must create an environment, a climate, in which he and his patient can tolerate the regression in a *mutual* experience" (p. 177).

In this image, psychoanalytic technique involves a sensitivity to the needs of the patient, such that these regressed parts, or self-states can find their expression. One needs to be mindful to not be too distant, which can be experienced as abandoning, or too close, which can be experienced as encumbering and intrusive. This is a *"mutuality"* which is governed by sensitivities to the patient's most intimate and complex needs. The developmental metaphor is inescapable here: Like a parent with a small child, the interaction is mutual, but is governed by sensitivity to the needs, limitations and tolerances of the child. Mutual but not symmetrical (Aron, 1996).

Within this unobtrusive and mutual relationship the patient will:

> find himself and get on with himself, knowing all the time that there is a scar in himself . . . which cannot be analyzed out of existence; moreover he must be allowed to discover *his* way to the world of objects – and not shown the 'right' way by some profound or correct interpretation.
>
> (Balint, 1968, p. 180)

This embodies a central contribution of the independent tradition of psychoanalytic practice, as described by Parsons (2009). Elaborating on Ferenczi's (1950) ideas of clinical process, Parsons emphasizes that:

> what comes from the patient, and what the patient experiences as his or her own discovery in the analytic encounter, matters far more than anything that comes from the analyst. What comes from the analyst is crucial, of course, but only for the way it facilitates patients' own experience of themselves.
>
> (Parsons, 2009, p. 223)

Thomas Ogden (2005) talks about the earliest holding that the mother offers the infant, that fosters the infant's sense of being alive, of "going-on-being," the sense that the continuity of being is sustained over time. This state is "subjectless," and asks of the mother an "abrogation of herself in her unconscious effort to get out of the infant's way" (p. 95). The mother's "*unobtrusive presence* provides a setting for the infant's constitution to begin to make itself evident, for development to unfold, for the infant to experience spontaneous movement and become the owner of their own sensations" (p. 95). Ogden suggests that if the mother intrudes herself as a subject apart from the reverie with the infant it will "tear the delicate fabric of the infant's going on being" (p. 94). "Unobtrusive" is not neutral or abstinent. Far from it: *It implies the very deepest engagement that is humanly possible.*

The analyst offers him or herself as "the human place in which the patient is becoming whole" (Ogden, 2005, p. 96). This type of holding is "most importantly an *unobtrusive state* of coming together in one place." (p. 97, emphasis added).

Often this involves interactions that do not feel anything like "psychoanalytic work." Winnicott talked about the patients who come in and tell about the details of their day or week as if that is all that is required, leaving the psychoanalyst feeling that no analytic work has been done; and Ogden describes conversations about art, sport, and other aspects of the patient's life with no interpretation of the content or commentary about the unfolding relationship. Far from being non-analytic work, these comprise the most profound human interaction, in their very ordinariness. In these "ordinary" conversations, we find the growth of the ability to derive thoughts from lived experience and the ability to dream, to process the raw data of experience into thoughts. The analyst's work, then, is to engage with the patient in these ways and to tolerate the feeling that no analytic work is being done. As Parsons (2009) adds, this involves much patient waiting on the part of the analyst.

The case of Kyle

Kyle has taught me how to be his analyst. Entering my office for the first time seven years ago, a tall, slightly chunky, and stylishly dressed blonde man in his twenties with thick glasses and an intense gaze, he stood in front of the couch facing me and then seemed to let his body fall into a sitting position on the couch. I understood that he inhabited his body and being in a very particular way, and figured that his body was already telling me a story of falling, of being dropped, and that much of our work and communication was going to be in the realm of physical sensation and action; his and mine.

His speech, very articulate and full of psychological insight, came at me like a pulse, an unstoppable tsunami of word-things. His words continued to come at and into me, sometimes slamming, sometimes penetrating, and sometimes caressing. Always totally physical. He told me that he was struggling with deep depression for which he had been in therapy since he was a teenager. He had just moved to be with his boyfriend and had ended a therapy of a few years which had helped him with procrastination while he had been in graduate school. In New York he had consulted with a few therapists and had yet to find someone with whom he felt comfortable. He told me that he was struggling with powerful feelings of hopelessness and familiar impulses to shut himself away in his apartment and withdraw from the world, something he had done repeatedly in recent years. He and his boyfriend of 7 years were fighting with increased frequency and their sex life had dwindled to almost no contact at all. His boyfriend had become very overweight, and neither seemed to be attracted to the other anymore. He was not working and was unsure what his next move would be. The boyfriend was independently wealthy and had a prosperous career, and Kyle experienced no urgency to find his own income. Kyle knew something was very wrong with him and his life.

Amidst the flow of words I gathered that when he would withdraw into himself, he would disappear into a timeless zone, a numb haze where he would become immersed in reading or the internet and would exist completely out of time, forgetting to wash, eat, or sleep. Hence the "procrastination" of his graduate studies.

At the center of his world was his mother. "She is a good person, but." He described her total involvement and impingement on his life. Most recently, via almost constant phone contact, she and her current husband had chosen all his graduate school courses and guided his day-to-day schedule and activities, although he attended school in another state. The relationship was laced with aggression and hatred and utter dependence. "She's a severe borderline personality disorder. It's all mood swings and tantrums," he said. He described screaming fights. 'When she flips, I flip." "The thing is, I love my mother, but I need time to myself. I need to make decisions, to motivate myself." When he had told her that he was in a relationship with a man, she had shown up the next day to intervene and to take him home. He resisted, but some months later he was duped into visiting home for a "family crisis." They trapped me, "which was OK, I guess: my life was going nowhere." He did subsequently reunite with his boyfriend.

I tried to get a grip on the narrative of his and his family's life, but, as was to become so familiar to me with Kyle, I'd become so flooded and confused that coherence was impossible. I did gather that his biological father had left his mother before he was born, that there had been some unsuccessful attempts at reunion, that he had been brought up primarily by his mother and her second husband, whom he also referred to as his "father," that there were two other major relationships in his mother's life. All these men were referred to interchangeably as "my father." His mother was one of ten Irish American children in a large, extended and alcoholism – dominated family. I could not sort out who were the mother's cousins and who the siblings; all were referred to as "my cousin," "my uncle," and so on, by Kyle. And to round things off nicely, some had the same names. Listening to all of this, I was imbibing the profound confusion that was the hallmark of his being. The closest and most meaningful relationship in his life seemed to be with his "grandparents." It took me some time to figure out that they were the parents of his biological father. Kyle made great efforts over time to visit and maintain a meaningful relationship with them.

I found myself continually confused. At first I panicked and would ask questions in a futile attempt to gain clarity, interrupting his flow of words. Explanations did not help. I learned that I had to settle into this felt world of confusion and near-psychosis, and somehow to find some way to get comfortable, or at least survive and keep my own mind intact. About a year into the treatment his "father" died of a sudden heart attack and I felt like I was falling into a deep pit, desperately trying to grab onto something to help me. Who, in fact, had died? For months he became embroiled in a lawsuit; he was the only beneficiary and there was a common-law wife who legally fought him and stole all the belongings from the deceased "father's" house. It did, eventually, become clear that the man who had died was his mother's first spouse after his biological father had disappeared from the scene. "We had a great relationship for a while," Kyle said, "We'd get high on pot together." My mind would scurry for a lifeline, a timeline. Hadn't this man been in his life when he was a young boy? They must have been getting high together when he was what? 11? 12? 13? "But," Kyle went on, "once the violence started things were never the same, and it never stopped." This father had systematically terrorized him and his mother for a number of years before finally leaving. The only relief had been getting high together. He was now inheriting some considerable amount from this man.

With nothing stable to hold onto in reality other than over-arousing intrusion, it was no surprise that he was sexually precocious and promiscuous from a very early age. He masturbated compulsively from age seven or eight. From age 14 or so he regularly had sex in public bathrooms with men. He describes being popular in those environments, where older men would perform oral sex on him or mutually masturbate. More panic on my part, as this world of abuse unfolded, but I did register that as he described sex, I felt that we actually had a subject, almost even a focus, and my mind could almost settle into a groove. Aha: an abuse narrative. This was, of course, the power of sex. He, as I, in these moments, could fleetingly feel oriented in a reality, in the space of the physical/sexual. As an adult his sexuality had been a zone of compulsion, psychological grounding, and mad manic omnipotence. He told me with a sense of jaded pride: "When it comes to sex and drugs, I've done everything. I've done every drug. Outside of dead bodies and children, I've done everything sexually." Indeed, he would go to great lengths to find an experience of ever increasing arousal: defecating in a man's mouth, watching a woman have sex with a dog, beating men on their testicles until they threw up in pain, are just some of the experiences he described. "I feel like god; I can treat a man like a toilet." "I am above the laws of reality. I can come while he throws up in pain. I am a god."

Degradation and control. No surprise, I felt coiled into this dynamic in the treatment. I drew attention to this. Was he not controlling and manipulating me, tying me up, in some kind of sadomasochistic relationship? I can't recall the exact words I used. But here's the point. He'd agree. Of course I am. This is me. What else would I do? I'd say "Can we examine this?" And of course he understood that this was what he did with people all the time, that it is what his mother and the "fathers" had done to him and that it was a repetition of unbearable trauma. To him, humdrum psychological insight. "Of course. I knew that." And he'd be off on some other narrative. More words coming at me. More experience, shit, flowing into me. Over time he did, however, recognize that this is why he has such difficulty with friendships. "I do see how I browbeat people. I just don't listen." He did dearly want to be more of a human among humans.

He became addicted to online sex. He'd create a persona for himself and disappear into an illusory world with various partners. "I can create myself in the persona of their ultimate fantasies."

I held on. Of course his dysregulation of time and space infused our work with increasing intensity. He'd miss appointments and offer no explanation. He'd call in for sessions sometimes on time, sometimes late. On numerous occasions I thought he had dropped out, only to answer the phone when it rang at the time of his session and hearing him start talking; no "Hello, this is Kyle," just picking up the session from where we'd left off some time ago. I was living in a world where one is continually forgotten and where one fears that everything can be gone with no reason or warning and where there are tears in the fabric of time.

He always paid for all scheduled sessions. The phone sessions became more bizarre and difficult to manage. A half hour into a session, he'd mention that he was driving in the car with his mother, or had a friend sitting next to him. He'd disappear for weeks and call, and only after a while mention that he was in Thailand or Indonesia with his boyfriend. No mention of whether he might have informed me. The prize goes to the session where I heard a persistent noise while we talked, and in response to my inquiry, he mentioned, "Oh, I'm in the shower." What country he was in? I didn't feel it really mattered at that point.

I tried to set some limits. More than with anything else, I was struggling with the unannounced absences. I addressed the issue and said that treatment required a more coherent structure, that he be present and at least give notice of his upcoming movements: seemingly ordinary boundary requirements. He was furious. The treatment almost ended. He was persistent and absolutely solid in his conviction. "That is your problem, not mine. This is me. I can't do this any other way," and so on. I was very affected by his rage with me. I felt deeply that I was in error to have tried to impose this structure on him, that it was my need to take back some power, some purchase on the out-of-control feeling that permeated the treatment. I could find no other thought in my head: He was right. This was about me, what I could or would not let myself tolerate.

It's so simple. Listen to the patient and be the analyst that *the patient needs you to be*. Not the analyst you think you are, or ought to be. I actually found this completely liberating. Was this masochism on my part, or "surrender" (Ghent, 1990)? Probably a bit of both, but once I allowed the experience in, and ceased trying to get him to talk about our relationship, to understand what was going on; once I allowed myself to flow with him, and "abandon any attempt at organizing the material," the treatment changed. In retrospect, I believe that his rage and insistence paradoxically provided a container for the treatment at that time, and enabled me to relax my own anxieties about his absences and dysregulation. Steven Cooper has offered insights about "mutual containment" in analysis (Cooper, 2000), and I believe that here we see Kyle protecting his own treatment and containing his analyst's fears, such that we and the treatment could thrive in his own idiom.

He had grown up, it emerged, with the persistent thought that he did not exist. Throughout his life he felt that he was a figure in someone else's dream, and that when they would wake up, he and all the world around him would no longer exist. He had grown up playing on the edge of existence: the sexual acting out, and hyper stimulation; an obsession with poisons – as a youngster he had elaborate plans to poison everyone he knew and had actually carefully made poisonous concoctions; and repeated experiences that he was not there. He said that he could differentiate what he called his dissociation and his not being there. Dissociation, for example, when faced with his "father's" violence, was out of fear and being overwhelmed. It was, according to him, soothing and sweet to dissociate, to feel nothing when beset by pain and terror. At least one is alive in order to dissociate. Most of the time he wasn't. He began to open his adolescent journals and we'd look at them in sessions. The sadness and constant longing to be dead. The daily onslaught of screaming fights and frequent violence. An obsessive interest in the Aztecs. They feared the sun wouldn't rise the next day, so they would make human sacrifices to the gods to be sure that the sun would indeed rise. Finally, this was him.

He never responded with much recognition to my comments that I now understood who he was and how he lived in this not-alive twilight zone – but then, almost nothing I said ever was, even though he would harangue me for my responses to him. However, more and more there would be sessions where he would make comments such as: "As I'm talking this is coming together, I can feel something." Of course, he was not going to take in from me. He had "to find *his* way to the world of objects" (Balint, 1968, p. 180).

There is much we can say about Kyle's developmental history to describe and explain his way of being in the world. Suffice it to say that I believe that the failures in holding and containing, along with the anni-hilating intrusiveness of his mother and the environment, kept from him the experiences that would have fostered an *existence*. He had no object or environmental constancy, and consequently could not trust that either he or the world would exist from one moment to the next. The treatment hinged on my being able to live with him in this ongoing non-existence and know it and tolerate it, and *expect no more*. In the words of Balint: "to create an environment, a climate in which" the patient and analyst "can tolerate the regression in a mutual experience."

Sessions were often filled with news items from the press and political discussions. He wanted to know my points of view on a variety of political and historical questions. The theme of much of the discussions was power, cruelty, and domination. He wanted to know about my family background, my family history. He became very involved with the Holocaust and read voluminously. I would speak openly and honestly to him. I left the question of the analyst's self-revelation many miles behind. I understood that he needed someone to partner with, to think with, to know, and be known by, in a non-impinging manner, someone with whom he could "dream himself into existence" in the words of Ogden (2009, p. 15). As Winnicott suggested, often these sessions did not appear to be anything like analysis or therapy. The crises of the Middle East, the Troubles Of Northern Ireland, the relationship between Russia and the Ukraine, the Chavez regime in Venezuela, and so on. On occasion he'd email me long essays that he'd written, or articles that he had found on the web, and he'd want to engage me in discussion about them. I would be with him in these discussions and only engage with the personal relevance to him on the rare occasions when *he* would offer it. For instance, he commented when talking about imperialism, that he understood now that his mind had been "colonized" by his mother's madness.

Generally, I was *unobtrusive* while being totally and intimately engaged. I'd silently make connections in my own mind to myself, tracking my reverie and my thought about his psychic process, while engaging in these discussions with sincerity and real interest. My strong feeling in these times is the opposite of what one hears most frequently, across psychoanalytic approaches: It is OK for these kinds of extra-therapy interactions or enactments to occur, as long as they are talked about or analyzed after. My feeling was that it was of the utmost importance that I enter these interactions as me, unadorned; and it was equally important, that they *were not* talked about after, unless *he* brought in the kind of connection such as the one I mentioned about his being colonized.

He was "dreaming himself into existence" with me. To play with Ogden's words, I believe my unobtrusive presence provided the setting for Kyle's constitution to become evident, for his development to unfold, and for his spontaneity to develop such that he became the owner of his own sensations. I believe I would have obtruded and diverted the whole endeavor by impinging my subjectivity unbidden by him: the part of me that needed to "analyze," "have good analytic sessions," to be a "subject" in an "intersubjective relationship" and to "resolve enactments." He had never had the experience of a mother who allowed herself the reverie of primary maternal preoccupation, wherein both the mother and the infant live in a co-constructed reality that is governed by the care and responsiveness to the infant's primary needs, and wherein the mother surrenders a part of her own orientation to the real world outside of their cocoon. Winnicott tells us the mother is in a kind of psychosis. I know what he means.

As with other patients like him, he would show rather than tell. He had liposuction surgery. He came to my office while still healing, peeled off his shirt to show me his torso, which had four small holes in, out of which oozed the last drops of the fat that had largely been removed. I stayed in the idiom of the moment. We talked about the liposuction treatment, the physical feeling of discomfort, and his wishes for a leaner body, his appreciation of the doctor, who helped him feel better without questioning his motives – he had not been that overweight. I held my thoughts about his showing me the embodiment of the damaged container of his mind, the ruptures in his psychic skin and in his reality, and his appreciation for me, that I was now meeting him where he needed to be met. In the language of Bion, we witnessed the introduction into the treatment of beta elements, "something more basic, more concrete and physical than what we generally mean by feelings" (Lombardi, 2007, p. 388). As Lombardi (2007) suggests, this process can only emerge within and through the actual physical bodies of the patient and the analyst. These elements, emerging via Kyle's body in the consulting room, were transformed, within my reverie and in the process of talking with him in his idiom, into the beginnings of alpha elements of more coherent experience.

He has begun to get better. The sexual compulsivity is a thing of the past. He looks back on this and can now talk about his desperate attempts to find contact and a sense of being alive. He has enrolled in a doctoral program in his field and, although attention is still an issue, is managing to get from one semester to the next. He ended the long-term relationship, realizing himself, that he felt abused and victimized by his partner's neglect and emotional abuse. He has actively impressed upon his mother and his step-father that they must be in therapy, and although this is hard going, and there are not great resources where they live, they are both being treated and the whole family scene has calmed down. He sets reasonable limits with them, and seems to appreciate how difficult it is for his mother, also, to be a human.

Most powerfully, he says that he is now alive and talks about never having felt like a living human among others before. He did not exist. This was most salient during the break up with the boyfriend which unfolded over a few years. On returning to the apartment they had shared to recover some belongings, some months after the break up, he found the now ex-boyfriend to have morphed into another being. He was now a thin man, his face altered by cosmetic surgery and the apartment transformed into a black-painted sadomasochistic dungeon. As Searles (1960) would say: "a non-human environment." He felt that the ex-boyfriend's metamorphosis not only revealed the boyfriend's true madness, but also served to illustrate the degree to which he, Kyle, had not existed, but had been a thing, using stimulation and perversion to construct a pretend dress-up version of being a human being. He thanked me. He was alive. We continue our work.

I offer my work with Kyle to illustrate that there are patients who can benefit from a wider range of relational practice. A technique that encompasses the ability to be unobtrusive while being related to the patient in the register and idiom that they require; a technique in which unobtrusiveness is not neutrality and in which enactments are to be lived with and through (Joseph, 1985), and not brought into the sphere of understanding or resolution, in which enactments foster the coming to life of the patient.

Regression, mutual regression, and regressive mutual regulation

Together with Kyle, I was able to "create an environment, a climate" in which we could both tolerate the "regression in a *mutual* experience" (Balint p. 177). Kyle could regress and bring in his deadness and not-yet-aliveness, and I found a way to tolerate the disturbances in the field of the analytic setting and in my own mind, so that this could to be a productive experience.

Regression is here not viewed as an artifact of psychoanalytic treatment, including the couch and the analytic setting, but rather as the emergence of the patient's inner world and his or her way of being in the world.

Etchegoyen (1991) puts it this way: "The patient *comes* with his regression, his illness is the regression" (p. 553). I would elaborate on this and say that the patient *is his regression*. Kyle *was* his regression, and by my being unobtrusive yet connected to him, he was able to *be* this Kyle in the treatment. Bromberg (1979) echoes this and suggests that when the analyst can be unobtrusive, the patient's regression:

> is something that will in and of itself occur under certain conditions, a primary one being that one allows it to happen. With many patients, in fact, I began to observe that the only way regression did not occur during the course of therapy was if I consciously or unconsciously prevented it by becoming increasingly interactional.
>
> (p. 651)

Aron and Bushra (1998) overview the concept of regression and reconsider it in the light of the contemporary relational emphasis on mutuality, and elaborate on Balint's idea of regression as a "mutual experience." They cast regression as the accessing of different states and underline that the most important aspect of the analytic situation is the facilitation of this access to altered states. Furthermore, they emphasize that this accessing of altered states is not and cannot be the property of the patient alone. There has to be a mutual regression, a mutual accessing of altered states. The analyst has to be available to enter and dwell in altered, uncomfortable, and sometimes traumatizing states, which may themselves elude description and elucidation. Acknowledging that my language is insufficient to describe the kinds of bizarre experiences I underwent with Kyle, I can say that feelings of catastrophic fragmentation, aloneness, uselessness, omnipotence, bizarre fantasies, and body dysmorphia were almost commonplace for me over a prolonged period of time. I would suggest that an insistence on intruding my own presence would have obviated the emergence of these phenomena in the analytic relationship and might have amounted to a version of Bion's "obtrusive object analyst" who would introduce interpretations to obviate being the receptacle for the psychotic parts of the patient's personality. I would add that introducing my own experience and pulling for a more mentalized and reflective interaction would have been an attempt to save me, not just from encountering the near-psychosis of Kyle's experience, but would also have protected me from the near-psychotic and fragmented states generated in my own mind.

For instance, I could have insisted on a more detailed description of his family relationships in order to clarify who was who. You will recall the chaos I experienced as Kyle described the various family members and "fathers." Perhaps one might have tried to build a genogram, formally or informally. This might have allayed *my* anxiety and confusion and might have brought coherence to the proceedings, and my notes. However, the "information" being conveyed was not simply the names and relations that comprised his family. Most importantly for our work, it was the sense of boundlessness, fragmentation, and absence of individual identity that was given to me, that I received, and then struggled to live within. When his "father" died, I lived through almost psychotic anxiety: ("Who in fact, had died?" see previously). This is a "mutual regression" (Aron & Bushra, 1998) that allowed me to deeply "enter his world" (Ellman, 1991) and "company" him (Khan, 1975).

The mutual regression required my availability to a mutual regulation (Stern et al., 1998). I adjusted to the unusual rhythms and outlines of Kyle's way of being. I had to tolerate his non-appearance in sessions, his bouts of incessant and pressured speech, and above all his unique signature and idiom that infused my mind and the total "field" of our work (Baranger & Baranger, 2009; Ferro, 1992). The mutual regulation that Stern et al. (1998) describe is always goal directed and in the service of growth. There were certainly large periods of time when I made myself available to be regulated in the direction of Kyle's internal world, his particular rhythms, and emotional cadences. This was a *benign regressive mutual regulation* where the "moving along" (Stern et al., 1998, p. 907) paradoxically involved a palpable loss of coherence and sense of direction on my part. But as Lachmann and Beebe (1996) suggest, it was this ongoing mutual regulation that was the therapeutic action itself, ultimately promoting the growth of Kyle's own sense of aliveness and self. Lachmann and Beebe (1996) also emphasize that these ongoing regulations between analyst and patient are internalized and ultimately affect the patient's own internal world and regulations "*regardless of whether they are ever verbalized*" (p.5, emphasis added). This, they suggest is the "therapeutic action of ongoing regulations" (Lachmann & Beebe, 1996, p. 5).

I found the uncertainty around Kyle's disappearances to be most unbearable for me, and when I tried to force him to adjust his behavior to fit with my psychological needs those feelings almost lead to a rupture in the treatment. Ghent's (1990) description of the experience of surrender, and his contrast of surrender with masochism, which he portrays as the perversion of surrender, was most useful to me in this work. To allow ingress to the patient's deadness and bizarre psychological life, to allow oneself to be a part of this regressive mutual regulation, one must surrender, and welcome these experiences that can take us far from our ideas of ourselves as analysts, and far from the ideal of the relational analyst-patient relationship.

Contemporary object relations and the unobtrusive analyst

The contemporary Bionians such as Ferro (1992, 2002, 2009) and Lombardi (2002, 2005, 2007) have helped us understand and engage with deadened, autistic-like states and breakdown in our patients. There is an appreciation of the analyst's participation in the construction of the field of analytic engagement, the use of the analyst's reverie as the pathway into the emerging narrative of the field, and the construction of narratives that "alphabetize" and make coherence (alpha function) out of the pieces of proto-experience (beta elements) that are often located in bodily sensations and symptoms (Lombardi, 2007).

For example, Ferro (2009) recommends staying as close as possible to the patient's own "narremes," "the various minor functional units" (F. Corrao quoted by Ferro, 2009, p. 46) that have the potential, via the containment process, to be united in a narrative with meaning. Thus, the patient's own story can be "opened up" (p. 6) and with the analyst's use of his own subjectivity and creativity, "original thinking" can begin. Very much in keeping with the image of the unobtrusive analyst that I am describing in this paper, Ferro recommends that the analyst not interfere with the patient's own story and use the "ingredients" and "worlds" (p. 6) that the patient offers. The analyst must not use "words that alter the patient's proto-narremes and do violence to them" (p. 6). He recommends that with patients that he describes as having "autistic tendencies" (p. 14):

> the analyst's contributions must be minimal so as to avoid administering doses of sensory or other stimulation that exceeds these patients' capacity to 'alphabetize' them. There must be no active interpretative activity centered on the patient's internal world or on the relationship, as the quanta of proto emotions aroused would give rise to their own immediate evacuation, given that the mind lacks the capacity to transform them into images emotions, experiences or thought.
>
> (p. 14)

ts that capture vividly those of this chapter. However, Ferro mmends that the analyst "has no choice but to act like a Greek i a Greek play, confining himself to commenting on the action that unfolds on the stage." This is where the conception of the unobtrusive relational analyst diverges. Certainly Kyle could not ingest anything offered to him, and I learned about his propensity to "immediate evacuation" of any elements that he was not ready to receive, and did not come from him. The image of the analyst acting like a Greek chorus commenting on the action on the stage conjures an analyst who is outside the interaction and can see it clearly. In a conception such as this, the patient must be available, interested in, and able to metabolize the ideas and observations of the analyst. The analyst's tool is interpretation above all else, even if it takes into account, with utmost sensitivity, the patient's readiness to ingest and stays as close as possible to the patient's own narremes and proto-mental activity. Certainly, Ferro's work is full of beautiful and evocative examples of the analyst's ability to play with the patient, to "stay as long as is necessary, with the manifest text" (p. 19) until the patient "has developed a gut, or mental function, capable of retaining, digesting and assimilating interpretations" (p. 19). I myself have metabolized much of this work and taken much clinical nutrition from it. I would add, though, that, again, the emphasis is on the analyst's interpretation as the ultimate tool of analytic healing. The analyst is described as lending his mind to the patient until the patient is able to metabolize interpretations. My approach places less emphasis on interpretations that *come from the analyst*, and places central importance on the healing power of the sharing and accompanying of the patient as the regressed states are entered. This foregrounds the accompanying and sharing of *states of being* and focuses less on the talking (interpretation) about what is happening or what has happened. Kyle, I contend, was helped to become alive, because he found someone who could accompany him in his deadness and terror, who could live through it with him and survive with him; someone who did not insist on imposing his own person/analyst and allowed Kyle to forge his own particular path to sentience and coherence: "to discover *his* own way to the world of objects" (Balint, 1968, p. 180).

Utilizing the work of Bion and the contemporary Kleinians, Riccardo Lombardi outlines the dense struggles within the analyst and the treatment relationship when working with people who are overwhelmed with shame, depersonalization, and psychosis (Lombardi, 2002, 2005, 2007). There is a focus on patients who do not experience themselves as located in their bodies or their own minds, and Lombardi offers feelingful descriptions of the analyst's physical response (Lombardi, 2005, p. 1092; Lombardi, 2007, p. 387) to the undigestible pieces of the patient's regressed experience and "modes of being" (Matte Blanco, 1988). Lombardi does emphasize the importance of the shared experience of these modes of being. However, the interventions that he describes involve the analyst explaining the ongoing experience in terms of the patient's internal world such that the patient can begin to occupy his or her own experience and discriminate self from other. These interventions may be contrasted with my work with Kyle, where rather than conveying understanding through spelling out what I believed was going on inside him and in the analytic field, I would engage with him in the very space that he was occupying, say, talking about the break-up of the Soviet Union. Yes, this kind of material suggests many interpretations of his internal world (the fragmentation that he may fear should he try to free himself from the tyranny of the colonizing internalized mother, and so on), or of our relationship (his wish and fear to take back his own autonomy and the terror that he would be left with new and pernicious persecutory objects that could infuse our relationship), but I would suggest that the "leading edge" (Miller, 1985) of these moments, to use Kohut's term, was the mutual engagement that Kyle was looking for as he worked with these issues in a symbolic register. My unobtrusive partnering with him allowed him to find his own way through these issues with the stability and holding of my company and emotional engagement. I would hold in mind the kinds of analyses explicated by Ferro, Lombardi, and others.

It seems to me that there are different ways to usefully understand the therapeutic impact of these discussions with Kyle. Certainly they could be said to involve the transformations of beta elements and that our relationship was providing the alpha function necessary for this. My observation was that Kyle was able to come together in aliveness in my engaged company, and was simply and explicitly not available for the ingestion of meta analyses of what was transpiring between us. One might also emphasize the function of implicit relational knowing and a process of fittedness between us that the Boston Change Process Study Group describe, and I'd like now to consider how the unobtrusive analyst might relate to these conceptions of therapeutic action.

Selfobject function, empathy, and the unobtrusive analyst

Certainly, there is much confluence between the conception of the unobtrusive analyst and the Kohutian idea that the analyst must be available for whatever "necessary but absent" (Lichtenberg et al., 1992) selfobject function the patient needs in the transference (Kohut, 1971, 1977), and must strive not to derail the development of that transference. Likewise, the self psychology emphasis on the careful use of empathy as a means of listening to and knowing the patient (Lichtenberg et al., 1984; Orange, 1995), the analytic couple's regulation of affect and arousal, the disruptions and repairs that comprise the treatment relationship (Lachmann, 2008; Stern et al., 1998), are all relevant to the formulation of the unobtrusive yet intimately engaged analyst that I am outlining.

Kohut, however, was skeptical about the ability of psychoanalysis to address patients who could not form stable narcissistic transferences and who exhibited "borderline" or "manic depressive" tendencies (1971, p. 18). He felt that patients who could not integrate their archaic exhibitionism and grandiosity "within the total structure of the grandiose self" (p. 18) would be unable to form the narcissistic transferences that constitute the curative factor in treatment. Accordingly, Kyle would not have been regarded as available for the kind of treatment that he and I built, particularly when we consider the degree of instability in his sense of self and other, together with his creation of the unusual treatment frame in terms of time and space.

In terms of the unobtrusive relational analyst, we find much in common with the work of the Boston Change Process Study Group (1998, 2002), who suggest that at times the change that occurs in analysis is not, and need not be, accompanied by explicit verbalization of the process. Lyons-Ruth (1999) suggests that implicit or procedural forms of knowing exist in "an implicit or enactive domain" and only emerge "in the doing" (p. 578). I would suggest that for Kyle, treatment could proceed only in a certain register: My thoughts about our process could not be made explicit, and instead we had to be engaged together in a certain form of "doing." For instance, when he showed me his punctured torso I stayed within the register and content that he occupied and talked about liposuction and his doctor, without any insertion of an understanding from outside of his immediate felt experience. I silently contained my intellectual and gut reactions to this moment.

Furthermore, perhaps the manner in which I allowed Kyle's disturbed inner world to manifest and fill up the treatment space between us and within me, can be fairly described as a form of empathic connection. This empathic connection involved little in terms of expressions of my understanding, but involved a growing implicit bond between Kyle and me that coheres with the caretaker – child "empathic connection" that Lichtenberg et al. (1984) outline.

If there is a divergence between this work and that of the intersubjective "friends of empathy" (Lachmann, 2008), I believe it would be in the area of technique and mutual regression: the allowing and holding of deeper and more disorganized states of being in the treatment. One might say that "moments of meeting" and "implicit relational knowing" are way-stations on the road to improved internal organization, integration, regulation, and relatedness. In the case of Kyle my "empathic connection" allowed him to bring his less regulated, less organized, less related states into the treatment and into my internal world. I believe I had to live through these *with* him and not do anything *to* him, in order for him to own the treatment space and shape it according to his own image.

Conclusion

I have described my work with Kyle to outline a contemporary reading and clinical utilization of the conception of the unobtrusive analyst outlined by Michael Balint (1968) and Enid Balint (1993). The related emphasis on the value of silence, waiting, and regression in a mutual experience are all seen as complementary to contemporary concepts of co-creation and the deep emotional engagement of the analyst with the patient in the analytic field. There is an emphasis on the analyst allowing for the patient's inner world to emerge within the analytic relationship in the idiom of the patient so that the patient can come to own their own sensations, body and mind. Particularly, but not only, with patients like Kyle who are not psychologically alive in a felt and recognizable way, the emergence of these regressed states often comes in the "enactive" register. I emphasize the value of the analyst allowing this process to unfold, to accompany the patient, and to not close it off with interpretations or investigations of the relationship that do not come from within the patient.

I have touched on some, but not all, of the influences from the contemporary psychoanalytic environment that are woven into my understanding of this feature of analytic process, and have tried to outline some similarities and some differences between this conception of the unobtrusive analyst and other ideas of clinical process.

Kyle was able to tell me that he felt alive for the first time in his life. He has continued to experience his own consciousness for the first time. He has described feeling peace in his mind, having clear thoughts, and listening and noticing others as having similar processes. He is excited and daunted by these seemingly simple everyday phenomena. He is still very much, and always will be, Kyle. As I write, he has begun to talk to relatives and intends to figure out a time-line of his childhood and his life. He would seem to have begun to discover his own subjectivity: his own "new beginning" (Balint, 1968, p. 131).

Note

1 I would like to acknowledge Dr. Donnel Stern, Dr. Sheldon Bach, and Dr. Bruce Reis for helpful comments in the preparation of this chapter.

References

Aron, L. (1996). *A meeting of minds: Mutuality in psychoanalysis*. Hillsdale, NJ: The Analytic Press.

Aron, L., & Bushra, A. (1998). Mutual regression: Altered states in the psychoanalytic situation. *Journal of the American Psychoanalytic Association, 46*, 389–412.

Bach, S. (1994). *The language of perversion and the language of love*. Northvale, NJ: Aronson.

Bach, S. (2006). *Getting from here to there: Analytic love and analytic process*. Hillsdale, NJ: The Analytic Press.

Bach, S. (2009). Remarks on the case of Pamela. *Psychoanalytic Dialogues, 19*, 39–44.

Balint, E. (1993). *Before I was I: Psychoanalysis and the imagination*. London: The Guilford Press.

Balint, M. (1968). *The basic fault*. London: Tavistock.

Baranger, M., & Baranger, W. (2009). *The work of confluence: Listening and interpreting in the psychoanalytic field*. London: Karnac Books.

Bass, A. (2009). An independent theory of clinical technique viewed through a relational lens: Commentary on paper by Michael parsons. *Psychoanalytic Dialogues, 19*, 237–245.

Bion, W. R. D. (1962). *Learning from experience*. London: Heinemann.

Bollas, C. (2009). Free association. In C. Bollas, *The evocative object world* (pp. 5–46). Hove: Routledge.

Boston Change Process Study Group, Stern, D., Sander, L., Nahum, J., Harrison, A., Lyons-Ruth, K., Tronick, E. Z. (1998). Noninterpretive mechanisms in psychanalytic therapy: The "something more" than interpretation. *International Journal of Psycho-Analysis, 79*, 903–921.

Boston Change Process Study Group, Bruschweiler-Stern, N., Harrison, A., Lyons-Ruth, K., Morgan, A., Nahum, J., Sander, L., Tronick, E. Z. (2002). Explicating the implicit: The local level and the microprocess of change in the analytic situation. *The International Journal of Psycho-Analysis, 83*, 1051–1061.

Bromberg, P. M. (1979). Interpersonal psychoanalysis and regression. *Contemporary Psychoanalysis, 15*, 647–655.

Bromberg, P. M. (1996). *Standing in the spaces: Essays on clinical process, trauma and dissociation.* Hillsdale, NJ: The Analytic Press.

Bromberg, P. M. (2006). *Awakening the dreamer: Clinical journeys.* Mahwah, NJ: The Analytic Press.

Cooper, S. (2000). Mutual containment in the analytic situation. *Psychoanalytic Dialogues, 10*, 169–194.

Ellman, S. J. (1991). *Freud's technique papers: A contemporary perspective.* Northvale, NJ: Jason Aronson.

Etchegoyen, R. H. (1991). *The fundamentals of psychoanalytic technique.* London: Karnac Books.

Ferenczi, S. (1950) *Further contributions to the theory and technique of psychoanalysis (2nd. Ed.).* London: Hogarth. (Original work published 1926.)

Ferro, A. (1992). *The bipersonal field: Experiences in child analysis.* London: Routledge.

Ferro, A. (2002). *In the analyst's consulting room.* London: Routledge.

Ferro, A. (2009). *Mind works: Technique and creativity in psychoanalysis.* London: Routledge.

Ghent, E. (1990). Masochism, submission, surrender. *Contemporary Psychoanalysis, 26*, 169–211.

Hoffman, I. Z. (2006). The myths of free association and the potentials of the analytic relationship. *IJP, 87*(1), 43–62.

Joseph, B. (1985 [1989]). Transference: The total situation. In M. Feldman & E. B. Spillius (Eds.), *Psychic equilibrium and psychic change: Selected papers of Betty Joseph* (pp. 156–167). London: Routledge.

Khan, M. (1975). Introduction. In D. W. Winnicott, *Through pediatrics to psychoanalysis* (2nd ed., pp. xi–xxxxix). New York: Basic Books.

Kohut, H. (1971). *The analysis of self: A systematic approach to the psychoanalytic treatment of narcissistic personality disorders.* New York: International Universities Press.

Kohut, H. (1977). *The restoration of the self.* New York: International Universities Press.

Lachmann, F. M. (2008). *Transforming narcissism: Reflections on empathy, humor, and expectations.* New York, London: The Analytic Press.

Lachmann, F. M., & Beebe, B. A. (1996). Three principles of salience in the organization of the patient-analyst interaction. *Psychoanalytic Psychology, 13*, 1–22.

Levenson, E. (1983). *The ambiguity of change*. New York: Basic Books.

Lichtenberg, J. D., Bornstein, M., & Silver, D. (1984). *Empathy I*. Hillsdale NJ: The Analytic Press.

Lichtenberg, J. D., Lachmann, F. M., & Fosshage, J. L. (1992). *Self and motivational systems: Toward a theory of psychoanalytic technique*. Hillsdale, NJ: The Analytic Press.

Loewald, H. W. (1980). *Papers on psychoanalysis*. New Haven, CT: Yale University Press.

Lombardi, R. (2002). Primitive mental states and the body. *International Journal of Psychoanalysis, 83*, 363–381.

Lombardi, R. (2005). On the psychoanalytic treatment of a psychotic breakdown. *Psychoanalytic Quarterly, 74*, 1069–1099.

Lombardi, R. (2007). Shame in relation to the body, sex, and death: A clinical exploration of the psychotic levels of shame. *Psychoanalytic Dialogues, 17*(3), 385–399.

Lyons-Ruth, K. (1999). The two-person unconscious: Intersubjective dialogue, enactive representation, and the emergence of new forms of relational organization. *Psychoanalytic Dialogues, 19*, 576–617.

Matte Blanco, I. (1988). *Thinking, feeling and being*. London: Routledge.

Miller, J. (1985). How Kohut actually worked. In A. Goldberg (Ed.), *Progress in self psychology* (Vol. 1, pp. 13–32). New York: Guilford Press.

Ogden, T. H. (1989). *The primitive edge of experience*. Northvale, NJ: Jason Aronson.

Ogden, T. H. (2005). *This art of psychoanalysis: Dreaming undreamt dreams and interrupted cries*. London: Routledge.

Ogden, T. H. (2009). *Rediscovering psychoanalysis: Thinking and dreaming, learning and forgetting*. London: Routledge.

Orange, D. M. (1995). *Emotional understanding: Studies in psychoanalytic epistemology*. New York, London: The Guilford Press.

Parsons, M. (2009). An independent theory of clinical technique. *Psychoanalytic Dialogues, 19*, 221–236.

Reis, B. (2010). Performative and enactive features of psychoanalytic witnessing: The transference as the scene of address. *The International Journal of Psychoanalysis, 90*, 1359–1372.

Reis, B. (2011, April). Silence and quiet: A phenomenology of wordlessness. Panel presentation at *Annual Spring Meeting*, American Psychological Association, Division 39, New York.

Searles, H. (1960). *The non-human environment: In normal development and schizophrenia*. New York: International Universities Press.

Slochower, J. (1996). Holding: Something old and something new. In L. Aron & A. Harris (Eds.), *Relational psychoanalysis, Volume 2: Innovation and expansion*. Hillsdale, NJ: The Analytic Press.

Slochower, J. (2004). *Holding and psychoanalysis: A relational approach*. Hillsdale, NJ: The Analytic Press.

Stern, D. B. (2004). The eye sees itself: Dissociation, enactment, and understanding. *Contemporary Psychoanalysis, 40*, 197–237.

Stern, D. B., Sander, L. W., Nahum, J. P., Harrison, A. M., Lyons-Ruth, K., Morgan, A. C. . . . Tronick, E. Z. (1998). Non-interpretive mechanisms in psychoanalytic therapy: The 'something-more' than interpretation. *International Journal of Psychoanalysis, 79*, 903–921.

Winnicott, D. W. (1958 [1965]). The capacity to be alone. In D. W. Winnicott, *The maturational processes and the facilitating environment*. New York: International Universities Press.

Winnicott, D. W. (1960). *Playing and reality*. London: Routledge.

Chapter 2

The flow of enactive engagement

This chapter will advance the idea that enactment can be regarded as a contemporary form of free association. Freud (1959b/1913) regarded free association as the key to a successful psychoanalytic process. Likewise, I conceptualize enactment as the key to the therapeutic action of a contemporary psychoanalysis. Freud (1959a/1912) recommended that the analysand say "everything that occurs to him without criticism or selection" (p. 112) and that the psychoanalyst should maintain a neutral position that allows these associations to flow freely without obstruction. Although we have traveled far from Freud's original suggestion of the abstinent psychoanalyst, I suggest that enactment, like free association, is a process that can be allowed to unfold freely by an unobtrusive yet deeply engaged psychoanalyst. It is this process that I term the "flow of enactive engagement."

I will recast free association as enactment that *happens* in psychoanalysis and fully involves both analyst and patient. The emphasis here is on things that happen in the course of a psychoanalytic treatment. I will draw on the ideas of the field of the analytic dyad from the River Plate group in South America, primarily Willy and Madeleine Baranger (2009) and their contemporary followers, such as Antonio Ferro (2002, 2009) and Claudio Neri (2009). I will suggest that enactments may be fruitfully conceptualized as the emergence of happenings or events in the treatment that narrate what is occurring in the field of the analysis. (I will elaborate on the conception of the field of the analysis below.) In short, both analysand and analyst participate in the field. They co-construct and are constituted by this emergent field. The field emerges as an entity in itself that is more than the sum of the two participants, rather like the "group-as-a-whole" (see as follows). The field can be thought of as the entity of the analytic relationship, which takes on a life and qualities of its own. The analytic pair comes to live inside this relationship or field. I will suggest that the advancement of the treatment process is best helped when the analyst recognizes the power of this emergent field or relationship and his or her role in it, and maintains an unobtrusive position in regard to that field's development. In other words, the analyst can allow the enactive field (Reis, 2010a), the "force field" if you will, of the analysis to unfold as its own narrative, without diverting it with interpretations or hurried explorations of "what's going on around here" (Levenson, 1989, p. 538). This approach can be regarded as addressing a register of treatment that is distinguished from that addressed by a more traditional Relational approach, which regards therapeutic process as the result of the continued analytic questioning of the nature of the therapeutic interaction.

Enactments are conceptualized as the emergence of regressed, unformulated (Stern, 1997), unconscious, and proto-mental (Bion, 1961) states of consciousness and states of being in the enactive field of the treatment. The flow of enactive engagement involves the surrender to (Ghent, 1990), and allowing of, states of mutual regression (Aron & Bushra, 1998) that involve both analyst and analysand. Often, these mutual regressions involve the emergence of self-states, worlds of feeling and sensation outside of awareness and inchoate. The work of the treatment is to allow the enactment to tell its story, to emerge in a fully felt way. This is the flow of enactive engagement and is, in essence, a mutual and creative act.

The analyst's participation in the flow of enactive engagement asks the analyst to carefully hold and contain the process as it unfolds, to be with the analysand, and to be mindful of not obtruding into this process. I borrow from the work of British independents such as Winnicott and Enid and Michael Balint in describing the stance of the "unobtrusive Relational analyst" (Grossmark, 2012) to flesh out this position. The analyst accompanies, even shares in, the journey that both participants take as the field unfolds and "tells its story."[1] Both participants look in the same direction, as it were. This expands the choreography of Relational psychoanalysis. Visually rendered, as well as facing and affecting each other, the members of this analytic couple sit side by side, facing the same direction, as the journey they create together carries them into new and heretofore unknown emotional and psychological territory.

From free association to the flow of enactive engagement

Freud regarded free association as the key mechanism by which the psychoanalytic cure proceeded (Freud, 1923a, 1923b), and he recommended that the analyst in no way interfere with this process. Echoing these sentiments, Christopher Bollas (2008) counsels us to not get in the way of the patient's free associations, to "not prevent free association from emerging" by being "overly active" (p. 19).

My suggestion here is that, likewise, the analyst not impede or obstruct the emergence of the flow of enactive engagement. In the classical tradition, free association was a mental activity that characterized the means by which the patient's unconscious was revealed in the analysis. I propose that the flow of enactive engagement with the patient's world allows the emergence of the most fragmented and inarticulable registers of the patient's psychic life in the analytic relationship.

I use the term "flow of enactive engagement," first, to evoke the independent tradition in which the analyst does not obtrude into the unfolding of the unconscious life of the patient, as captured by Balint's (1968) description of the unobtrusive analyst; second, to shift the therapeutic action away from the mental, one-person connotation of free association;[2] and, finally, to foreground the enacted and enactive process in which the analyst must accompany the patient (i.e., to be fully engaged while being unobtrusive). For patients who have no words for their inner life or who are inhabited by self-states that defy verbal description, classical verbal free association may not provide access to these inchoate inner worlds and states. Words may be regarded as acts among other acts that emerge in the analysis. For many patients, such as I will describe later, words and associations function as things to be experienced by the analyst rather than associations to be followed for their denotative meaning. They can "tell" their lives, however, and their pain and psychological make-up in their own idioms of *action* and *engagement*, idioms that are joined by the analyst, who is ready and available to live with and through (Joseph, 1989) these self-states and mutual regressions.

The flow of enactive engagement evokes the involvement of both analyst and analysand. Bollas (2009) reconsidered free association and suggested a "free talking" patient in the presence of an analyst who employs "evenly hovering attention" (Freud, 1923a) or "free talking" (Bollas, 2009). In addition to these images, I see a patient who, unable to verbally narrate his or her experience, engages in a "free being" or "free becoming" within the environment provided by the analyst. The analyst listens with his or her full experience, emotional, physical, intellectual, always partly conscious and always unconscious, always both present and partly dissociated. It is an enactive engaged experience, a process that the analyst simultaneously gets out of the way of and with which he or she is completely engaged.

A brief etymological investigation of the term "free association" would seem to evoke some of these ideas. Bruno Bettelheim (1982) changed our understanding of Freud with his careful analysis of James Strachey's translation of Freud in the *Standard Edition*. Bettelheim offers us fresh insight into the meaning of some of Freud's key concepts. Among the concepts that came under his scrutiny is free association. He points out that, on occasion, Freud used the word *einfall* (e.g., Freud, 1925) and that Strachey always uses the term "free association" as a translation. Bettelheim notes that *einfall* means allowing something to spontaneously come to one's mind, as in "it happens to occur to me" (p. 96). He suggests that this word contains a more fully psychological meaning than the purely mental meaning of the "incorrect" term, free association (Bettelheim, 1982, p. 94). Free association, according to Bettelheim, invokes a more conscious and "logical" (p. 95) process, whereas *einfall* suggests a more spontaneous occurrence. Bettelheim suggests that this spontaneous process is more closely connected to the "unconscious from where this idea suddenly emanates" (p. 95).

In fact, the word *einfall* has more to offer us. It also contains the word *falle* (to fall). To have a thought, then, evokes a thought *falling* into one's mind. And, the sense of mutual enactive engagement evokes a hidden sense that has lain like a sequestered self-state, tucked away inside the concept of free association: a mutual state of falling or a falling together. This sense of falling – into something with a patient as both patient and analyst regress together in the emergent field, and the more disturbed and damaged parts of the self emerge in the treatment – is a common experience.

Einfall, therefore, evokes many images of mutual falling: into altered and deeply regressed states of being; the Freudian fall from secondary to primary process; from ego to id; the philosopher Hans-Georg Gadamer's concept of falling into a conversation together (Gadamer, 1965, quoted in Stern, 2010); and the fall into the altered state of sleep. Jean-Luc Nancy (2009) observes that "by falling asleep, I fall inside myself" (p. 5) into deep solipsism. And to sleep is to dream. Ogden (2009) suggests a process of "talking-as-dreaming" as "the place where analysis occurs" (p. 14). This is an area of overlap where the patient's and the analyst's dreaming occur together. Talking-as-dreaming is talk in analysis that is infused with primary process thinking, the thinking that goes on with no "understanding work" (Sandler, 1976, p. 40). The patient free associates and the analyst accompanies with his or her own "waking dreaming" or reverie, which involves a surrender to one's own primary process experience. These are the analytic conversations, which often do not seem to comprise analytic work, yet move in the direction of helping the patient become more alive and more human (Ogden, 2005).

The concept of the flow of enactive engagement, then, includes the experience of falling together into the dreamlike primary process of the patient's free talking, along with the analyst's reverie, and adds a dimension of engagement in enacted experience. The sediment of cumulative relational trauma may not come into the analytic space via free talking and associations, but via the actual happenings and doings of the analytic relationship; it can only come through unmentalized and "undreamable" (Ogden, 2009, p. 16) occurrences that involve patient, analyst, and the dyad's unity, the field.

I must note, however, that the flow of enactive engagement does not imply that the analyst enters the patient's world and the emergent field of the analysis, and takes leave of his or her own abilities to think and process the experience. Like the analyst's reverie or evenly hovering attention, it suggests an altered state that exists simultaneously with other states. It also asks that the analyst be clear and firm around boundaries while allowing for the inevitable ambiguities and challenges that, when one connects with these areas of functioning, occur as part of the treatment.

The "Field" of a psychoanalysis

There has been renewed interest in the work of the River Plate Group (e.g., Brown, 2010; Stern, 2015; Zimmer, 2010). In a series of prescient articles, Madeleine and the late Willy Baranger (2009) – French analysts who settled in Uruguay after time in Buenos Aires – outlined the theory of the "field" of an analysis. Suggesting that the field is comprised of the conscious and unconscious realms of both analysand and analyst, they proposed that in every analytic relationship both participants develop powerful unconscious fantasies of the nature of the dyad as it unfolds and

the nature of the cure that is wished for and feared. At any gi
the analyst can understand what is happening in the treatm
to the current state of fantasies about the relationship. The
been adapted and expanded by many contemporary writers,
Ferro (1992, 2002, 2009), who provides numerous examples of how he
understands the treatment process in terms of a constant message from the
unconscious of the dyad as to the state of the relationship. The message
comes from the field, rather than from either participant.

The piece of the Barangers' contribution that is most relevant to the
suggestion I am advancing here is that the field – constituted by both participants' conscious and unconscious fantasies and fears, their worlds of
internal object relations and the transferences that ensue – develops and
takes on a transformative and generative quality of its own. Narratives and
worlds are generated that are more than the sum of their parts (i.e., the
internal and intersubjective worlds of the patient and analyst).

On the face of it, this is a phenomenon with considerable validity. Who
has not registered that a relationship can develop a quality or color that
is more than the contribution of the two members? It is commonplace to
experience oneself as living *inside* a relationship that pulls and pushes
one into a particular self-state or way of being as if it has a mind of its
own. From my own perspective, as a psychoanalyst who practices group
psychoanalysis as well as individual treatment, the theory of the field is
organic and coherent. The group therapy community has, for many years,
paid attention to the idea of the phenomenon of the group-as-a-whole
(Agazarian, 2006; Anzieu, 1984; Bion, 1961). The group-as-a-whole has
its own presence and is more than the sum of the interpersonal and intersubjective relationships in the room. Indeed, anyone who has been a part
of a large crowd or mob will attest to this phenomenon. Some group therapists, such as Agazarian (2006), confine their interventions to talking to
the group-as-a-whole and only address individuals as a container or "role"
for a piece of the group-as-a-whole's dynamic.

I believe that these ideas find much coherence in the Relational literature, particularly in the work that Steven Mitchell (1988, 2003) was
advancing: That is, we do not find the unconscious inside the mind of one
individual even as he or she interacts with another, but rather the unconscious emerges in the field that is generated in the interaction and unfolding of the treatment. The ideas of the field or the dyad-as-a-whole can be
said to expand these ideas. Certainly, there is much resonance here with

recent theorizing about the "analytic third" (Aron, 2006; Benjamin, 2004; Ogden, 1994). Space does not allow for a more thorough discussion of these concepts.

The unobtrusive relational analyst, the field, and the flow of enactive engagement

In Chapter 1 I outlined the position of the "unobtrusive relational analyst." I suggested that the silent or quiet accompanying of a patient has erroneously been conflated with classical ideas of "abstinence" and "neutrality." I argued that for patients whose subjectivity and internal object worlds are damaged and distorted as a result of developmental trauma, failure, and pathological identifications, engagement by the analyst as an independent subject may be premature. Such patients may seek – and need – to relate from a more regressed self-state, dominated by more primitive states of merger, dependence, and lack of self/other definition and object constancy. The analysis may be best served by an analyst who remains unobtrusive and allows the patient's internal worlds to dominate the scene. The analyst must accept that words are empty and "abandon any attempt at organizing the material" (Balint, 1968, p. 177). The analyst creates "an environment, a climate, in which he and his patient can tolerate the regression in a *mutual* experience" (p. 177; emphasis added). The regression is mutual but not symmetrical (Aron, 1996). This mutuality is governed by the analyst's sensitivities to the patient's most intimate and complex needs, and, like a parent's attunement to the needs and tolerances of a young child, is deeply intimate. In this "environment" the patient can come to his or her own sensations and mind in the connected presence of the analyst. Hence, unobtrusive is not neutral, but deeply intimate and engaged.

The unobtrusive analyst may wait quietly and patiently, or be engaged and lively. The key is that the analyst is joining the idiom and rhythm of the patient and, therefore, allows the patient to inscribe the treatment with his or her own psychological signature. The analyst accompanies the patient in this process, much like a child analyst will accompany the patient who brings in a toy and wishes to engage in play together. The emphasis here is on the quality of "with-ness" (Reis, 2010b, 2011). Many of our most troubled patients had parents who simply could never be with them in any meaningful manner as their lives and experiences developed. When we are *with* these patients but do not try to do anything to them, we create the possibility of a "new beginning" (Balint, 1968), and provide the ballast that the ensuing journey may require.

Thus, the unobtrusive relational analyst allows for the emergence of the patient's inner world, but not simply as a solitary phenomenon. In an unobtrusive manner, the analyst participates in the field of the analysis – indeed cannot not participate in it – and allows the field to unfold and tell its own story: A story that cannot be known until it emerges. The analyst is unobtrusive yet deeply involved in the flow of enactive engagement that takes the analysis on its revelatory journey.

The following is a brief description of my work with Ruben, which I hope illustrates these concepts in action.

The case of Ruben

Ruben is an American man whose father was a Brazilian immigrant. He is a big, handsome, South American man who speaks in a strong, resonant voice, and who carries himself with an air of familiarity and confidence. The patients whom I see before and after him have remarked on his regular salutations: "Hey! How are you?" and so on. One supervisee wondered if he was a friend of mine due to this air of ownership and comfort in the waiting room. He dresses in beautiful clothes that often leave me envious, and more important, he wears them with ease. He will often enter carrying a half-smoked cigar – he will stub it out before entering the building – and on one occasion, proclaimed with beautiful timing: "Doctor: Sometimes a Cigar is Just a Cigar!!" From the get-go, there has been so much to potentially comment on, interpret, and consider with him. I have done little of this: The overriding message from Ruben is that he needs to dominate the treatment space and me; he quickly let me know that he is not interested in taking much from me. He seems, however, to deeply need me to join with him, to enjoy, admire, and accept him.

Here we go! This is the beginning of the flow. The flow and the field of ongoing enactive engagement. To ask him to consider the nature of our engagement – "what's going on around here?" – would, I believe, damage the potential for this flow to take us somewhere new.

From the beginning, Ruben has enjoyed engaging with me outside the confines of therapy talk. Quickly gathering that I am British, he has shared his great love of soccer and his devotion to one of the teams from the English league. Of course, as luck would have it, his team is the deadly enemy and rival of the team I have followed with boyish enthusiasm since my youth, and we've made no secret of our rivalry, often engaging in playful jousting and ribbing each other. Unfortunately, my team is in a 30-year slump whereas his team is in the ascendancy; thus, much of this humor is at my expense. But, it really is a hoot, and I look forward to these moments of fun during the bleak and trying times with him.

Of course, Ruben's bigness and dominance might be regarded as an exemplar of a phallic narcissistic structure – his big voice and big presence. He drives a white Hummer! He told me exactly why he needed a BIG CAR when he made the purchase: "Because I'm BIG; that's why!" And there's the massive roaring lion tattooed across his chest that he removed his shirt to show me. Of course, he has a huge and powerful physique – he works out regularly and intensely – that he displays by the way he dresses.

Nonetheless, my experience of Ruben and of these big and potentially intrusive qualities is not one of menace, avoidance, or aggression. Rather, it seems to me that he is engaging, seeking, "probing" as Emmanuel Ghent (1990) would have said. Neither interpretation nor exploration of our relationship would have been acceptable to him; it would have created a distance between us that would have left him wanting in ways that he may not have been able to articulate. My interest was in being *with* him and finding out where we were going.

Ruben grew up with his father. The story was that his mother died when he was an infant. His father, recently emigrated from Brazil, only had a short time with her before her death. Ruben has few memories of his first decade – just a sense of deep longing and shame, and the perceptual, hallucinatory image of ragged, rusty iron and steel: old, rusty, hard, unfriendly, and toxic. Having finished high school, he worked in his father's construction business. The proximity to his father was poisonous for him. He was continually verbally and emotionally assaulted by his father, called a "good-for-nothing" and far worse. His father was particularly adept at assaulting his manhood, always insulting him as weak, stupid, and ineffective – using the kind of language we can easily imagine (e.g., "You'll never amount to anything").

Ruben was, unsurprisingly, shy and withdrawn as a child, living in constant anxiety and with a continuous sense of self-loathing and worthlessness. He found it impossible to make friends at school and in the neighborhood. His father had no sense or connection to who his boy might be beyond some kind of extension of his own narcissistic self. Thus, Ruben found no connection to others and none to himself. He had no clue what he might want to do, who he might want to be. To stick his head up, to be his own person and have his own desires, was too dangerous.

After his father died, Ruben took over the business and, shortly thereafter, received an unannounced visit from . . . his mother. She told a long, shocking, and confusing story. His mother said she had a short affair with Ruben's father in New York and had lived with him beyond Ruben's birth. When their relationship became strained – both were young, overwhelmed, and not very responsible – Ruben's father threatened her so violently that she ceded custody of her boy to the father and left New York to live a carefree fitness and recreation-oriented life far away. Only now, with a heavy heart and much regret, she was looking for Ruben. She also had some undefined hope to reconstitute a family that now included a grown brother and sister, fathered by different men, for Ruben to get to know.

So, on the advice of his girlfriend, Ruben came to treatment, as he struggled with a roller-coaster of feelings and moods. He was confused, angry, and resentful with the world: with a mother who had abandoned him to an abusive father and with a father who had withheld from him the only thing he had ever wanted but could not articulate. Not only that: He was angry and resentful with himself for not having listened to his own sense, time and again, that his mother was somewhere, close at hand, and not dead as he was told.

Rage. Of course, it was coming. Over time, I heard more and more about altercations in stores, arguments with friends and rumbles in clubs. He took up boxing and described some vicious and painful bouts. And then we are in it. Five years into treatment, clean from years of domination by addictions to cocaine, alcohol, and sex, and gradually establishing a sense of continuity and trust in others, including working on relations with women, he goes into father-assault mode. It is 2010. "Obama is the worst president in the history of this nation. . . . We need another Bush. Now there was a great man." And on he spews. I simply can't take it. As an argument, I quote the Nobel Prize-winning economist who supports Obama. Things get worse. It feels all kinds of ugly. He sneers at my suggestion that there is racism behind the Republicans' all-out attacks on Obama (like his father, Ruben is a Black man). Eventually, we look at each other, squared-off, full of rage: boxing. "You don't fight fair!" he cries. And, I realize that I have hurt him. I could not have believed such a thing was possible. We talk more. Not about what all this means psychologically, but just talk. He tells me how shamed he felt when I quoted Nobel Prize winners. "Where d'you learn that?" he asks. I talk. Bullied by a bigger and stronger older brother who could pin me down, I learned to use my mind, be a wiseass. Outsmart him. I tell him this, and how I tried so desperately to cover my hurt. He tells me about experiences, primarily with his father. It is all about domination and submission, being done to or doing to another. This is how he was taught to know and feel another's presence and came to feel alive himself. And, now, we feel more alive. If the lie that he had grown up with was that his mother was dead, the lie that had infused the treatment was that the treatment was totally alive. Alongside the great improvements in the course of treatment was a deadened self-state, a not-dead and not-alive internalized mother. The only way to aliveness was this: beating each other, and surviving.

The fantasy of the field, of the nature of our relationship – that aliveness comes through this kind of emotional pugilism – could only come through our living through it together. No examination of our relationship, no interpretation of his aggressive altercations, could have taken us to the anguish of trying to find life in pain, abrasion, and poison. I came to *share* this with him, to accompany him in this prison, and I do believe he felt it. The fight had to come. The field took us there, and somehow we were in it. Both of us were regressed, both conscious and unconscious, and both were trying to stay afloat, hoping the ballast of years of productive work together would be strong enough to hold us.

Thankfully, our ship does not sink. New winds now blow us into the territory of love. He does not know what that is. He hangs his head and grieves. He just doesn't know what that feels like. Never has before and feared he never would. And, I try to be with him and let it be. I know that he is a tender man trying to be alive. I don't say much and he keeps coming and we keep working. He sends me a postcard from his vacation, to the effect that the ocean never lets you down, it goes on and on. When we resume after the summer I do not interpret this or offer a suggestion about how this relates to our relationship: I do not suggest that he is discovering object constancy in the form of the "primary substance" of the ocean (Balint, 1968, p. 70). Instead, I respect and allow the field and the flow of this engagement to continue to tell our story. Indeed, it is the flow of enactive engagement.

Notes

1 We are accustomed to speak of "narrative" or the "telling of a story" as a product of language and interpretation in psychoanalysis. The idea here is that a

story is told in the events, interactions, affects, and states that emerge in the analytic couple. These may or may not be given form via subsequent interpretative reflection. We might say that the enactment itself *is* the interpretation. See Chapter 7 for a fuller discussion of this concept.

2 See Hoffman (2006) for a critique of the classical concept of free association.

References

Agazarian, Y. (2006). The invisible group: An integrational theory of "group-as-a-whole." In Y. Agazarian (Ed.), *Systems-centered practice: Selected papers on group psychotherapy* (pp. 105–130). London: Karnac Books.

Anzieu, D. (1984). *The group and the unconscious.* London: Routledge.

Aron, L. (1996). *A meeting of minds: Mutuality in psychoanalysis.* Hillsdale, NJ: The Analytic Press.

Aron, L. (2006). Analytic impasse and the third: Clinical implications of intersubjectivity theory. *International Journal of Psychoanalysis, 87*, 349–368.

Aron, L., & Bushra, A. (1998). Mutual regression: Altered states in the psychoanalytic situation. *Journal of the American Psychoanalytic Association, 46*, 389–412.

Balint, M. (1968). *The basic fault.* London: Tavistock.

Baranger, M., & Baranger, W. (2009). *The work of confluence: Listening and interpreting in the psychoanalytic field.* London: Karnac Books.

Benjamin, J. (2004). Beyond doer and done to: An intersubjective view of thirdness. *Psychoanalytic Quarterly, 73*, 5–46.

Bettelheim, B. (1982). *Freud and man's soul.* New York: Knopf.

Bion, W. (1961). *Experiences in groups.* London: Basic Books.

Bollas, C. (2008). *The Freudian moment.* London: Karnac Books.

Bollas, C. (2009). Free association. In C. Bollas (Ed.), *The evocative object world* (pp. 5–46). New York: Routledge.

Brown, L. J. (2010). Klein, Bion and intersubjectivity: Becoming, transforming, and dreaming. *Psychoanalytic Dialogues, 20*, 669–682.

Ferro, A. (1992). *The bipersonal field: Experiences in child analysis.* London: Routledge.

Ferro, A. (2002). *In the analyst's consulting room.* London: Routledge.

Ferro, A. (2009). *Mind works: Technique and creativity in psychoanalysis.* London: Routledge.

Freud, S. (1923a). The libido theory. In J. Strachey (Ed. & Trans.), *The standard edition of the complete psychological works of Sigmund Freud* (Vol. 18, pp. 255–262). London: Hogarth Press.

Freud, S. (1923b). Psycho-analysis. In J. Strachey (Ed. & Trans.), *The standard edition of the complete psychological works of Sigmund Freud* (Vol. 18, pp. 235–254). London: Hogarth Press.

Freud, S. (1925). Negation. In J. Strachey (Ed. & Trans.), *The standard edition of the complete psychological works of Sigmund Freud* (Vol. 19, pp. 233–240). London: Hogarth Press.

Freud, S. (1959a). Recommendations to physicians on the psycho-analytic method of treatment. In J. Strachey (Ed.), *Collected papers* (Vol. 2, pp. 323–333). New York: Basic Books. (Originally published 1912)

Freud, S. (1959b). Further recommendations on the technique of psychoanalysis: On beginning the treatment. In J. Strachey (Ed.), *Collected papers* (Vol. 2, pp. 342–365). New York: Basic Books. (Originally published 1913)

Gadamer, H. G. (1965). *Truth and method*. London: Continuum.

Ghent, E. (1990). Masochism, submission, surrender. *Contemporary Psychoanalysis*, *26*, 108–136.

Grossmark, R. (2012). The unobtrusive relational analyst. *Psychoanalytic Dialogues*, *22*, 629–646.

Hoffman, I. Z. (2006). The myths of free association and the potentials of the analytic relationship. *International Journal of Psychoanalysis*, *87*, 43–61.

Joseph, B. (1989). Transference: The total situation. In M. Feldman & E. B. Spillius (Eds.), *Psychic equilibrium and psychic change: Selected papers of Betty Joseph* (pp. 156–167). London: Routledge.

Levenson, E. A. (1989). Whatever happened to the cat? Interpersonal perspectives on the self. *Contemporary Psychoanalysis*, *25*, 537–553.

Mitchell, S. (1988). *Relational concepts in psychoanalysis*. Hillsdale, NJ: The Analytic Press.

Mitchell, S. (2003). *Relationality: From attachment to intersubjectivity*. Hillsdale, NJ: The Analytic Press.

Nancy, J. L. (2009). *The fall of sleep* (C. Mandell, Trans.). New York: Fordham University Press.

Neri, C. (2009). The enlarged notion of the field in psychoanalysis. In A. Ferro & R. Basile (Eds.), *The analytic field: A clinical concept* (pp. 45–80). London: Karnac Books.

Ogden, T. H. (1994). The analytic third: Working with intersubjective clinical facts. *International Journal of Psychoanalysis*, *75*, 3–19.

Ogden, T. H. (2005). *This art of psychoanalysis: Dreaming undreamt dreams and interrupted cries*. London: Routledge.

Ogden, T. H. (2009). *Rediscovering psychoanalysis: Thinking and dreaming, learning and forgetting*. London: Routledge.

Reis, B. (2010a). Enactive fields: An approach to interaction in the Kleinian-Bionian model. Commentary on a paper by Lawrence J. Brown. *Psychoanalytic Dialogues*, *20*, 695–703.

Reis, B. (2010b). Performative and enactive features of psychoanalytic witnessing: The transference as the scene of address. *International Journal of Psychoanalysis*, *90*, 1359–1372.

Reis, B. (2011, April). Silence and quiet: A phenomenology of wordlessness. Panel presentation at *Annual Spring Meeting*, American Psychological Association, Division 39, New York.

Sandler, J. (1976). Dreams, unconscious fantasies and "identity of perception." *International Journal of Psychoanalysis*, *3*, 33–42.

Stern, D. B. (1997). *Unformulated experience: From dissociation to imagination in psychoanalysis*. Hillsdale, NJ: The Analytic Press.

Stern, D. B. (2010). *Partners in thought: Working with unformulated experience, dissociation and enactment*. New York: Routledge.

Stern, D. B. (2015). *Relational freedom: Emergent properties of the relational field*. Hove, New York: Routledge.

Zimmer, R. (2010). A view from the field: Clinical process and the work of confluence. *Psychoanalytic Quarterly, 89*, 1151–1165.

Chapter 3

Psychoanalytic companioning

Introduction

> *what if I wanted to be whole? If I wanted to work with the darkness rather than against it?*
>
> —(Matthew Sanford, 2006, p. 128)

This quote was written by Matthew Sanford. At age 13 his family's car skidded off the road while he slept in the back, killing his father and sister and leaving him paralyzed from the chest down and confined to a wheelchair for life. In a moving and thoughtful memoir (Sanford, 2006) he spells out the years of psychological and physical suffering that followed and the many harrowing treatments he underwent, ultimately finding healing and renewal through the practice and eventual teaching of yoga. I found much that is stirring and evocative in this memoir, especially his gradual realization that the traditional treatments he had initially undergone were oriented too exclusively to what had been lost and to overcoming the trauma too quickly. He spins the following metaphor that captures the transition in his awareness of what was needed:

> Imagine walking from a well-lit room into a dark one. Imagine the darkness as a visual expression of silence. My rehabilitation made a mistake with the silence by focusing on the absence of light. It too quickly accepted the loss and taught me to willfully strike out against the darkness. It told me to move faster rather than slower, push harder rather than softer. It guided me to compensate for what I could not see.
>
> (Sanford, 2006, p. 127)

He describes the treatment that eventually helped him accept the loss of his legs and the "compensation" of his arms and his wheelchair to carry him through life. He felt that he was not whole, and gradually, with much help, began to contemplate a new form of wholeness that encompasses his losses, the darkness, and the absence of his legs (and his father and sister):

> But what if the darkness (the silence) is a fundamental part of us, of our consciousness? How do we overcome an essential part of who we are? For me . . . working against the silence deadened my sense of living and accelerated a negative sense of death.
>
> (p. 128)

Matthew Sanford needed someone to go further *into the darkness with him*, rather than simply pull him into the light. His brave and insightful journey recalled for me the painstaking and painful work we engage in with our patients who have suffered massive, cumulative, and relational trauma, leaving them constricted and tortured in their internal worlds and in their relations with others and with reality. His memoir captures a simple idea that is at the heart of this book: that true healing often involves going further *into* our patients' worlds of suffering and private madness rather than working to move them *out* of these states. In this paper I address how one works intersubjectively and authentically as a relational analyst with patients and states where there is no mutuality and no differentiation of self and other, when consciousness is dominated by part-object relatedness and fragmented, constricted, and bizarre experiences of self, other, and the world and where symbolization and reflective function are greatly limited (Director, 2009, 2014; Grossmark, 2012a, 2012b; Reis, 2010a, 2010b, 2011; McGleughlin, 2011). I will foreground the utility of imbricating the ideas of object relations theory together with relational conceptions of clinical interaction such that patients and self-states that are unavailable for dialogic connection can be reached and engaged with. Much as Matthew Sanford (as noted earlier) so eloquently described the value of entering into the darkness rather than rushing into the light, I will offer a register of relational psychoanalytic engagement, wherein the analyst companions the patient into the dark, "archaic" areas of functioning and regressed object relations that are not available for discursive interaction or mutual study, rather than seeking to foster greater relatedness and mutuality in the session.

Object relations theory, regression, and the unobtrusive relational analyst

Of all psychoanalytic theories, object relations theory has consistently addressed more primal and less developed forms of relatedness, psychic structures, and ways of thinking. There has been a sustained interest in patients who can be said to not live in the world of whole objects, whose internal world is dominated by paranoid-schizoid functioning and defenses (Klein, 1946), whose development, or at least parts of it, were characterized by disobjectalization (Green, 1999), the failure of pleasurable and attuned engagement with primary others, and the lack of adequate containment and holding, such that experience of self and other and internal objects themselves are not developed and defined. The patients and these states can be said to be dominated by the psychotic part of the personality (Bion, 1957). Sadomasochistic object relations predominate relatedness and space, time and continuity of self are compromised. Winnicott has so memorably alerted us to the patients who have not developed a comfortable and sustained sense of going-on-being and who thus have difficulty separating waking from sleeping, alive from dead, and inside from outside (Winnicott, 1945). These are patients and self-states where there is a paucity of the ability to symbolize, mentalize, and to represent. Winnicott (1945) described such patients as being in "bits and pieces" (p. 150) and Sheldon Bach focused on patients with greatly compromised reflective function and reflective self-awareness, who have limited coherence or continuity of self over time (Bach, 1994, 2006) and suffer ongoing experiences of emptiness and the fear of relational impingement (Bach et al., 2014). Such patients do not "learn from experience" as Bion would say (Bion, 1962). It would seem that the relational trauma suffered by these patients was cumulative and early, affecting critical periods in the development of relatedness and intersubjective maturation. Recent work by (Levine et al, 2013) and Botella and Botella (2004) has widened the appreciation of areas of functioning that are beyond representation and the manifestations of absence and negative space in the clinical relationship.

In terms of clinical practice, the Kleinian tradition has tended to rely almost exclusively on interpretation by a neutral analyst and while embracing the value of countertransference and containment, has generally placed the analyst as able to comment from outside of the interaction. Mitchell highlighted the inherent contradiction in such an approach that views the patient as dominated by early paranoid-schizoid dynamics, yet relies on an integrated and coherent patient to work with and utilize the analyst's interpretations about that very process (Mitchell, 1997). Yet as has been stated, such patients also pose a dilemma for relational theory and practice, where there is much focus on the real relationship and mutuality between patient and analyst.

However, there is also a tradition of finding other ways to be clinically helpful to these difficult-to-reach patients. Writers from Ferenczi onward have struggled with the technical challenges of engaging with these more archaic, traumatized, and less developed states. As described in Chapter 1, Michael Balint talked of patients who required a relationship that was "more primitive than that obtaining between two adults" (Balint, 1968, p. 161). Writing in the psychoanalytic tradition that celebrates the clinical value of benign regression in treatment, he suggested that when the analyst can abandon the need to interpret and relate to such patients and can allow him or herself to be utilized as a primary object or a primary substance (p. 69), the patient can regress to the area of the basic fault within themselves and, together with the analyst, facilitate a "new beginning." Balint saw that these patients were unable to utilize the predominant psychoanalytic treatment of his time that relied so heavily on interpretation as the prime agent of therapeutic action. I suggested in the foregoing Chapters (Grossmark, 2012a, 2012b) that such patients also have great difficulty utilizing the contemporary focus on mutuality in the analytic relationship and that a treatment that emphasizes the patient's participation in understanding the interaction in the here-and-now can foreground the self-states of the patient that are more psychologically developed and related and can overlook the areas and self-states of the patient that are not organized around coherent object relatedness and representation.

Working in the tradition of the "elasticity of psychoanalytic technique" (Ferenczi, 1928) and influenced by Balint (1968) and Slochower (1996, 2006), I outlined in Chapter 1 the concept of the "unobtrusive relational analyst" (Grossmark, 2012a) who need not obstruct the unfolding and emergence of the patient's idiosyncratic internal world in the treatment, yet remains emotionally engaged and intimately connected with the patient. I suggested that the analyst can allow a process wherein the patient and analyst enter into regressed and unformed states that "cannot and perhaps should not be put into words" (Balint, 1968, p. 174), and not intrude upon this process by discussing it with the patient. I proposed that the analyst "listen to the patient and be the analyst that the patient needs you to be" (Grossmark, 2012a, p. 637). The register of psychoanalytic companioning described in this chapter continues this work.

Psychoanalytic companioning

Winnicott has famously described how the infant gradually understands that he or she and the mother have an inside and an outside. With this development comes the sense of relationships between whole persons and the comprehension of external reality. The patients I am thinking about here have trouble in this very area. They are not able to "have relationships between whole persons" (Winnicott, 1945, p. 148) and engaging with them as if they can, runs the danger of compounding a false self adaptation to the world – often the very reason they have come for treatment. What I want to highlight is Winnicott's description of how the mother and infant engage with each other such that the infant can develop the sense of self and other, and of reality itself. The mother's breast and milk, he says, do not come into meaningful relation with the hungry infant until "the mother and the child *live an experience together*" (his emphasis). The mother shows tolerance and understanding and hence produces a situation that, with luck, will promote the "first tie the infant makes with an external object" (Winnicott, 1945, p. 152). We can take from this that the patient and the analyst, like the mother and the child, cannot find each other and come into "relation with each other" in a nurturing helpful union until they "*live an experience together*" and it is this mutual experience that fosters the "first tie to an external object," that is, relatedness. Moreover, it is via this mutual experience that the infant begins to relate to external reality.

In Winnicott's schema the comprehension of external reality is gained by the mother's allowing the infant to create an illusion that he or she has created the breast/mother. When the mother's wish to feed a hungry baby and infant's need to feed – "overlap there is a moment of illusion – a bit of experience which the infant can take as *either* his hallucination *or* a thing belonging to external reality" (p. 152). The mother does not challenge the infant's hallucination. She "enriches" the hallucination and thereby gives the infant the illusion that external reality corresponds to his or her own capacity to create. In this way the infant connects to and develops an alive experience of self in relationship to an other.

In a related vein, Botella and Botella (2005) have also outlined the developmental necessity of the hallucinatory function that underlies the development of internal objects and the perception and experience of external reality. Likewise, Ferro and Civitarese have described the emergence of the hallucinatory field of the treatment that both patient and analyst inhabit together (Civitarese, 2013; Ferro, 1999, 2002).

I take from this that the analyst must be prepared to live in the world of illusion with the patient and *not* intrude the coarse reality of the external world or of the "reality" of the relationship. From the infant's position, and indeed from that of many of the patients I am talking about:

> the object behaves according to magical laws, i.e. it exists when desired, it approaches when approached, it hurts when hurt. Lastly it vanishes when not wanted.
>
> (Winnicott, 1945, p. 153)

It seems to me that Winnicott is valuing the states of psychotic unintegration that characterize the infant's early life. They have their place in normal development and likewise they also have their place in psychoanalytic work with primitive patients and less troubled patients who enter into regressed states. To me, his ideas seem to support the sense that we must allow the work to enter the darkness, the states of unintegration, and not hurry the patient out of them.

When such states of unintegration emerge, it can appear that the patient is not engaged in treatment, perhaps asking for concrete advice, missing sessions, rarely showing any interest in talking about themselves and certainly not the analytic relationship. There is often an inability to adhere to the common frame and contracts of treatment regarding time and space. It certainly can feel as if the whole treatment situation is subject to "magical laws" and illusion and the analyst most commonly feels "taken for granted," if not outright offended and enraged. At times it can feel as if the patient is not in treatment at all. Such patients offer a challenge to all psychoanalysts, and perhaps especially to a relational approach that values the intersubjective and mutual aspects of the clinical interaction. Rather than seeing such patients as not engaging in treatment, or as not involved in relatedness and dialogic interaction, from this perspective, we can consider that the patients are in fact deeply involved in the treatment, in ways that they cannot possibly know for themselves, let alone describe in words.

They show rather than tell. I would suggest that they are conveying the need for a particular kind of object relationship, that, when engaged with *on its own terms*, may both tell the story of their developmental trauma and offer a way into their own inner world such that the pain that they have yet to experience can become available for psychological work.

Inner regulation of the body and of the self comes from the parents accompanying the child, sometimes actively and sometimes quietly and softly. Didier Anzieu (2010) has mapped out the growth of the "skin ego" and describes how the way the infant is positioned and held enables the child to experience a surface, to be alive and connected, and have a center of gravity. The tactile along with the parents' vocalizations and the music of accompaniment regulate and locate the child.

These ideas from psychoanalytic theory cohere nicely with the many observations of children and their caregivers in the child development literature.

Colwyn Trevarthen (2001) draws on a multitude of studies to illustrate the ways that mothers and infants mutually regulate and join together in what he calls a "joint consciousness in companionship" and "cooperative intersubjectivity" such that the infant learns what it is to be a "person in relation to others" (p. 112). This seems to harmonize so well with Winnicott's observations. There is an emphasis on the vocal and rhythmic companionship between mother and infant. Daniel Stern (1993, 2010) talks of "relational emotions" that anticipate contingent rhythms and sympathy from others; Trevarthen (2001) talks of the rhythmic mirroring of vocal and gestural expression, Tronick (2001, 2003) describes a "dyadic state of consciousness" between mother and infant, and Brazelton (1993), some years back, had observed "proto-conversations" of rhythmic vocal mirroring and expressive movements.

Infants, Trevarthen observes, develop social awareness and meaning in purposive action primarily by *sharing* and *companioning* with their carers. He makes a clear statement:

> Contrary to the old view that human social awareness is mediated by instructive and corrective actions of adults who are intending to constrain impulsive self-serving actions of children, new value (is) given to a *primary sharing of subjective impulses* behind conscious experience and intentions.
>
> (Trevarthen, 2001, p. 101)

In other words it is the sharing and *being with* infants in the rhythmic, vocal, and motoric registers that enables them to grow as humans, not the telling them how to be. Here I recall Winnicott's perspective that reality and relatedness are gained by not intruding upon the infant's illusion, but by the sharing of experience.

I would suggest that here we find an outline of the companioning register of psychoanalytic engagement. When we are working well with a patient, there is implicitly a sense of rhythmic synchronicity and mutual affective regulation and containment. When working with regressed states these features of companionship, proto-conversational and rhythmic engagement are foregrounded. When the verbal is stripped of its meaning, we are left with the vocal. The sound, harmony, and rhythm predominate. It is our work to stay as attuned as possible to the patient in this register and to not ask him or her to shift to a more verbal and intellectual register. Even when a patient is in the verbal/intellectual register, it is often the vocal and rhythmic domain that holds the affect and potential engagement. As Trevarthen and Winnicott have suggested, it is via this sharing and companionship that the human learns to be a "person in relation to others," not through instruction or via thinking about it. More recently, Bruce Reis has extended these concepts from infant research to adult psychoanalytic treatment, describing the shift in focus from knowing (interpretation) to the lived experience of sharing and affect and has written of the importance of the analyst's position of "being-with" patients as an essential "with-ness." Change, he suggests, is not a function of mutative interpretation or a knowing about what had occurred in the patient's past but about "an intersubjective experience at the limits of understanding" (Reis, 2009, p. 1370). In a related vein, Black (2003) has described the largely non-verbal mutual sharing of energy between patient and analyst in co-constructed enactments and has argued for the value of leaving such enactments in the realm of the unsaid. What follows is an account of psychoanalytic companioning where "joint consciousness in companionship" (Trevarthen), "living an experience together" (Winnicott), and "working with the darkness rather than against it" (Sanford) helped the patient gain a greater connection to his inner and outer reality and to the world of relatedness.

The case of Bernard

Bernard first came to see me five years ago. He was in his early forties and in his own words "wretched" and "lost." He was disheveled and unshaven, easily mistaken for a homeless person. He was one of two identical twin boys employed in the family's very successful manufacturing business. The aging father ruled the family and the family business with a volatile and iron fist and it was always assumed that both sons would simply follow in his footsteps and run the business. Bernard barely ever showed up for work in the business, drank too much, rarely left his small, messy apartment, and spent many days alone, drinking, masturbating, and watching TV. He was clear that "I *could* do things, but I just don't," "I'm frightened to grow up." He described a desultory life of following various passions of his: video games, politics, music, and his various pets, but was very aware that he was not truly living a life. He aimed much venom and loathing at his father who he described as terrifying and dominating him and his whole family. He regarded his mother as totally "desiccated" by the father's domination and offering him very little. No one in the family or his world seemed to understand him and why he was so unable to simply "do anything." He immediately related to me via the objects of my office: the bits and pieces of me, if you will. He spoke admiringly of my pen, the pieces of art in my office, the plants, and my shoes. He moved around the office removing various crumpled pieces of paper, used tissues, keys, phone, and so forth from his pockets, placing them on various surfaces during the sessions. He would adjust his clothing sometimes undoing his belt and zipper to re-adjust himself, all the while talking and seemingly unaware. He would move and fiddle with the ornaments, furniture, cushions, and plants in the office. I felt that I was being shown that he was, as Winnicott, would say, "in bits." He told me about a video game image that involved a space-man shattered into small pieces. His mental process was similarly fragmented. While clearly possessed of great verbal ability and erudition, pieces of stories, of his life, of his moment-to-moment emotion came out in a scattered and unformed manner. There seemed to be little thread to his wanderings and any questions I asked would often be met with a frustrated "hold on: wait, wait, let me just say" and he would continue on his meandering path. Certainly, I was being shown how it was that he couldn't get anything done in life, but more profoundly I felt drawn into this fragmented, unformed world where continuity and cohesion were but abstract concepts and where I too was not experienced as a whole person. This, it seemed, was what "unintegration" looks like. In Bion's language, a world dominated by beta elements with little alpha function or containment. Within myself, I would become similarly fragmented in sessions, often losing track of the substance of what was being talked about and frequently unable to recall what we had just been saying.

Emotionally he was as disorganized and disrupted as his speech and thought. He conveyed wild impulsivity and volatility, showing great sensitivity and tenderness, as well as vicious and savage rage. When rageful he would actually bare his teeth and literally snarl. His rage scared me. His sweetness touched me. But this form of relatedness could not be called empathic or connected. The displays of rage and wildness seemed to me to be happening in my presence rather than involving me. I seemed to barely exist for him outside of what Winnicott described: I existed when desired, I approached when approached, I hurt when hurt, and I vanished when not wanted.

In keeping with this he would show up when and how he needed, sometimes missing sessions, mostly late by 15, 20, even 40 minutes, and often seemingly unaware that I was trying to end the session at the end of the hour. His sense of time, his sleep-wake cycle, appetite, self-care, and his sense of space and location were often quite distorted and dysregulated. He could go for days without sleep, and on occasion would wear the same clothes day and night for many days without changing or showering. During these periods he certainly could have been taken for an itinerant and mentally ill person. He was in fragments and not located in himself. He knew that he always sought to twin with others, and could evoke a sensation of deep connectedness with people, as indeed, he did with me. I was reminded of a comment Winnicott made about the loss of integration of one identical twin. I quote:

> The localization of self in one's own body is often assumed, yet a psychotic patient in analysis came to recognize that as a baby she thought her twin at the other end of the pram was herself. She even felt surprised when her twin was picked up and yet she remained where she was. Her sense of self and other-then-self was undeveloped.
>
> (Winnicott, 1945, p. 149)

Bernard described he and his twin as "womb mates." Growing up, they would often be confused with each other even by his parents and grandparents. Of his relations with women, which had been fleeting, intense, and never sustained, he said "I melt with them: I twin and fuse." On one occasion he told me in great detail about a pair of artists who had attained notoriety by literally merging into the same person via a series of plastic surgeries that altered their faces and bodies until they were identical. His relating-through-fusion was clear from early on. I think he felt comfortable after our first few sessions and wanted to tell me that he liked me. What came out of his mouth was: "I wanna be you." How can you like someone if there is no defined you and other? So "I like you" simply becomes "I wanna be you." It obliterates both parties.

We spent much time talking through the weekly, even daily crises, of his volatile life, but I found myself calmed and grounded by the idea that the bigger picture here involved a process of self-definition and integration. I also began to work with the idea that the treatment would most beneficially proceed in the registers of *his* experience; the vocal, the rhythmic, motoric, and tactile, and that my work would be to accompany him in a kind of "consciousness in companionship" (Trevarthen, see previously) rather than trying to change or intellectually explain him or interrupt his flow to ask for any reflective function. Indeed, he told me "please, for god's sake, don't summarize me." Inquiries into his experience or any attempt to interrupt his world and introduce self reflection were met with an almost incredulous look, as if to say "Come on: we're not going to do *that* now are we!", and he would resume his flow.

He had been in various treatments previously and said that he had gained much from some of these experiences, particularly where he had felt taken care of and mothered. He had also attended a well-regarded day treatment program in the city for some time and had been thrown out because of his volatile rage and the threat of violence. The violent rage had apparently also made his prior treatments difficult to sustain, and on more than one occasion the therapist or analyst had ended the treatment.

All his life he had found ways to be damaging to his body and his mind. Cavalier drug use as a teenager was accompanied by wild fights. He always ended up on the receiving end of a beating. In college he collapsed while high from a vicious cocktail of alcohol and drugs and fell from a great height. He required extensive surgery. He courted all kinds of physical disaster. He engaged in frequent violent fights, suffering numerous injuries, and he showed me his arms and torso that were an archipelago of scars. Rage would come like a tsunami and there were various assaults in bars and at the family factory leading to violent punch-ups and worse. He was prone to road rage of course and I became numbingly familiar with his treacherous journey to and from his family business via the bridges and tunnels. Arrests were not uncommon as were nights in the "Tombs." The family's lawyers would be called in to sort things out.

He would describe horrific violence in his dreams and fantasy life and would take me into gut-wrenching discomfort. In particular I recall his vivid versions of how to kill in hand-to-hand combat that he had read about online. Leaning in to me so close that I could smell his breathe and baring his teeth he emphasized the need to twist the knife in the gut after piercing the skin. Moments like these would really take me "into the darkness" with him, and again, I did not experience this violence as directed at me, so much as a plea to accompany him in this state. This was the darkness and desperation that accrues when access to the mother's mind is foreclosed. Force and torture are the only options.[1] Most alarming was a family fight at a gathering that involved him physically assaulting an older male cousin. They had to be pulled apart and the police called.

I was certainly very scared myself by his violence, but was paradoxically helped when he told me that as a young child he and his brother would play the "pain game." He would have his brother hit, pinch, and, on occasion, burn his arms and legs with a lighter. My thought was certainly that love and death, pleasure and pain were tragically joined for him, a not uncommon feature for people who are not differentiated, but also that pain and violence might be attempts to separate, to feel something that could be called his own. Bernard told me: "It's such a lovely pleasure to fuck myself over, to squander myself." "Violence is liberating. Suicide and murder are the ultimate liberation."

The courting of physical pain is often a last ditch attempt to find the outline of one's physical body when the holding of infancy has been such that the psychic skin (Anzieu, see previously) has not formed sufficiently. This is the most basic level of self-definition.

In my work with Bernard I was unobtrusive yet very engaged. I did not structure him beyond the beginning and end of sessions and payment, and allowed him within sessions to take us wherever his flow took us. I'd work as calmly as possible with him on whatever he brought in. I believe we created a space within which we could float and he could come to himself. I would join whatever and wherever he took us, in a felt, mutually regressive way. What I said would embellish his images and flow, rather than speak from outside of his experience, as I internally strove to find a place for whatever disturbing experience or altered state was growing inside of me. During the first years of our work, these states were chiefly ones of fusion and fragmentation. I recall feeling unfathomable dread and terror for my own sanity when at one point I found us dressed identically and I had the sensation that my voice and body were changing into his. In moments such as these I was entering the darkness with him rather than fighting against it, to echo Matthew Sanford. There were many registers to the mutual regressions. An unobtrusive relational position does not only mean quiet, patient waiting. This is not a question of withholding one's subjectivity, but the provision of a particular register of subjectivity. In time he would evoke songs and movies that I was often familiar with. We would look at You Tube videos together, and often sing songs as he recalled one band or another. As frightening as some of the violent and sadistic regressions were, these shared moments of song and laughter were joyous and tender. The thing is, we were in the shared accompanied register of the tactile, mobile, and vocal, rather than that of verbal and intellectual. We were enjoying our "joint consciousness in companionship" and "sharing of subjective impulses" in proto-conversations (Trevarthen). He would bring me food and drink. We'd snack together. He would send me music via email, links to books, films, and articles he liked. I'd read them. I did not regard these as assaults on the boundary of treatment, did not attempt to interpret, and did not engage in consideration of what may be going on between us. I did not confront his absences or lateness. I did not want to stand outside of these experiences, of the illusion, and comment on it. To try to make "material" out of this kind of engagement is to lose it, to do damage to the nascent moments of self-other definition and the comprehension of external reality that were beginning to grow. Recall Winnicott's ideas that the comprehension of external reality and the other's subjectivity comes not from the interjection of reality that breaks the illusion, but by enriching the illusion and living within it. And in these and many other ways, we have lived many hours of illusion and even hallucination together. This is the companioning register of the engaged but unobtrusive relational analyst. Bernard seemed to comprehend and appreciate this. For alongside such intimacies as sharing songs from our younger years, he would be assiduous that I not reveal anything at all about my actual personal life. (I should add that for me this was all very evocative. I grew up sharing a room with my brother who is 15 months older than I. We'd spend countless hours sharing activities and being intuitively in contact. While not twins, we certainly shared consciousness, and later we also had to, literally, fight our way to separateness.)

Certainly, I had to manage volatile aggression and destructiveness in the sessions. Bernard would often throw a stinging barb at me as he was leaving. "You analysts are all such assholes" or some anti-British slur. I took it that he experienced the end of the session as a physical hurt. To speak of aggression is too organized a concept. His struggle was with a raw destructiveness (hence the bared teeth) that would destroy himself and those around him: a mutually assured destruction. I would let him know that he had hurt me but did not interpret that he found the end of sessions painful: He knew that. Again, I did not experience these attacks as really hurtful, rather as a yearning for a space where such aggression could be both real and not real, i.e., a transitional space. One day after many such stings he re-opened the door, leaned in, and said: "Why do I do that?' "Why do I want to hurt you?" "I must want you to throw me away like everyone else did. Don't throw me away. Please."

Four years into this four times per week work, he came into the session and seemed unable to decide what he wanted to communicate. He shrugged and wordlessly groaned. I groaned back in a similar idiom. He vocalized a kind of "now what"? noise. I responded with a vocalization. He vocalized anger. I did too. And on we went for a good 15 minutes just making noises together. At moments it was really quite funny, and I think we were quite delighted with ourselves for being so creative. But amazingly we also made noises of sadness and hurt, and he and I evoked real emotions. He talked about a piece of sound-art, an installation that featured a speaker that emitted diffuse sounds. He mimicked these "voice waves." He told me that there is a part of Grand Central Station downstairs near the Oyster Bar, where, if you stand in one corner and someone stands in the opposite corner, you can whisper and the other person can hear you clearly despite all the hubbub of the concourse. The ceiling is shaped in a certain way that carries the sound. We continued to make sounds with each other. Our sounds seemed to become more mournful, deeper, more basso, and one of us – I don't remember who (no surprise) – said that this was like whales communicating under water. We looked at each other as we both had the same realization: We had created an amniotic environment and we were twins, wordlessly connected through the waves. I believe that this is going *into* the inner world, the darkness, with the patient in mutual regression, as opposed to commenting on and striving for understanding from the *outside*. It is psychoanalytic companioning.

So, gradually Bernard has begun to appreciate his place in external reality and to feel that others are separate and have their own subjectivity. In amongst his flow there were images of re-birth, of escapes from subjugation, the attainment of independence and waking up. One day he said: "I live in such a small narrow, interior world. Others explore the world around them." There were gathering images of pieces coming together. He remarked one day that walking across the park he had suddenly realized that the different areas of the park, that had always felt like separate, not connected places, were actually part of one whole park and were easily accessible, one from the other. His emotional volatility calmed slowly. He sang a song called "High, Low and In-between". He talked of spacemen surviving the heat of re-entry intact (recall the shattered video-game spaceman from his initial sessions).

He surprised everyone when he leapt at the chance to take an underdeveloped branch of the family business and develop it when they were about to off-load it. Ignoring his father and brother's predictions of disaster, he proceeded and he continues to be committed to it.

Most telling is that he is now quite different to sit with. He rarely moves around the office fidgeting and fumbling. He piles his belongings neatly and he talks in a calmer, much more coherent manner. Emotionally, the manic, horrifying sadism rarely appears and he talks openly about his own fear and his vulnerability with people and work. A space for thinking has developed inside his mind, and hence impulses can be mediated, contained, and symbolized.

He has a girlfriend. They have dated for eight months. As one might predict, it's been a roller coaster, and they drink too much, but he talks of her with great tenderness and tries to take her feelings, her emotional reality into account. It doesn't come naturally for him. He has developed some ability to reflect on himself and his destructiveness. He talks about his fear that he can destroy the relationship with his girlfriend and his business, and wants me to help him manage that.

Just this week he said to me: "We do our best in here when we don't talk about anything. Just music. We riff. Love. I feel I can live."

I think that Bernard is finding a "new form of wholeness," to quote Matthew Sanford. One that is truly his and which encompasses the many damages he has suffered over his life. He is getting there with me companioning him, into both the darkness and the light of our "cooperative intersubjectivity."

Psychoanalytic companioning, intersubjectivity, and the patient's internal world

I suggest that my work with Bernard highlights the psychoanalytic work that can be accomplished when companioning patients in the dimension they inhabit: the dimension of primal affects, primitive object relations, motility, and proto-experience. Bernard did not want to be "summarized" and mostly only wished for me to exist as a figure in his hallucinatory world of illusion. The suggestion of this chapter is that by entering into this world with him, I fostered the creation of a space within which the processes of self and self-other definition, and the recognition of reality could take hold. It is my contention that he was not available to hear anything from his analyst that came from outside of his own world of illusion and omnipotent control. Paradoxically, I would argue that in receiving his silent need for an object relationship "more primitive than that obtaining between two adults" (Balint, 1968, p. 161), I was able to offer my subjectivity in a dimension that he *could* use.

I wonder if the way we have talked about using and offering the analyst's subjectivity in the relational literature has too often emphasized the knowing and exploratory aspects of one's subjectivity; the expression of subjectivity that aims to help develop the dialogic and reflective aspects of the patient. Our case studies are replete with accounts of the resolution of enactments after an insightful and sincere expression of the analyst's understanding of what has transpired in the treatment relationship and a case study of mine would be a case in point (Grossmark, 2009). I am suggesting here that there are many other registers of the analyst's subjectivity that the analyst can choose to offer in the course of treatment and there are treatments with the kinds of patients that I am describing where a different register of the analyst's subjectivity is required. They may not be exploratory, but I would argue that they are certainly expressions of the analyst's subjectivity. The register of unobtrusive companioning in mutual regression involves the presence of a subjectivity whose signature is surrender (Ghent, 1990), responsiveness, receptivity, and unknowing.

It also occurs to me that when companioning Bernard into his world, I seemed to be in a liminal world that simultaneously embraced his private and deeply personal inner world as well as the world of reality and engagement. Relational writers have recently engaged with the previously perplexing question of private internal spaces in relational psychoanalytic theory and practice (Bass, 2014; Cooper, 2014; Corbett, 2014; Harris, 2014; Seligman, 2014; Stern, 2014). Corbett comments on the relational credo that "we are none of us one" and worries that

> all of this relating . . . places an untenable demand on both patient and analyst alike, and risks crowding out the dreamy leisure of reverie and co-creation of a fantastic life through which the patient and analyst may come alive as otherwise.
>
> (Corbett, 2014 p. 640)

I would suggest that in letting Bernard's internal world of primal object relations find it's full expression in the treatment relationship, there emerged a "fantastic life" in which he came alive as never before, even if this particular reverie was a little more nightmarish and percussive, rather than one of Corbett's "dreamy leisure." This would seem to illustrate the unobtrusive relational analyst at work, simultaneously unobtrusive to the process, or third, that is emerging while engaging deeply with the register and idiom the patient brings. This often requires a protracted ability to not know or pre-empt where this enacted narration will take us. As Donnel Stern comments: "To be engaged is not necessarily to know the nature of that engagement" and "usually the best I can do is stay out of its way" and "attend as closely as I can to recognizing whatever is arriving in the range of my knowing" (D. B. Stern, 2014 p. 680). These are all statements of the analyst's subjectivity that tilt toward the receptive and unknowing register, very much in keeping with the idea of psychoanalytic companioning.

Psychoanalytic companioning and the dimensions of intersubjectivity

Lecours and Bouchard (1997) outlined a map of the "dimensions of mentalization." Borrowing from Bion they suggest that mentalization involves the transformation of raw excitations and sensations into meaningful experience. They suggest different modalities or channels of expression of experience that increase in complexity and integration from somatic and motor activity to imagery and verbalization. All of these levels correspond to different degrees of internal containment, which is to say that *all* of these modes involve the transformation and elaboration of raw proto-experience into psychic contents: All are modes of thinking. I take from this that even when a patient is in the somatic mode or the motor mode this itself is a form, albeit less elaborated, of mentalization, of thinking. For Lecours and Bouchard "such 'poorly' mentalised events are thus welcome occurrences in analysis" (p. 865). Hence Bernard's motility, apparent disorganization, and volatile affect need not be regarded as the absence of mentalization, but rather as his own unique "dimension of mentalization," that asks to be recognized and companioned with *as such*. I would argue, and indeed always felt, that he was doing psychoanalysis, but doing so in the dimension that was true to the experience and level of mentalization that he lived within. Indeed, Lecours and Bouchard suggest "that each patient displays certain specific emotional 'dark zones' (*no less*) that are less mentalised and others that are more mentally elaborated" (p. 871), but all are modes of transformation and can thus be regarded as thought and communications.

I would suggest that the shape and texture of the field of the treatment, the third, is shaped to a large degree by how the patient and analyst think, that is, the dimension of mentalization that predominates at any given time. The texture and quality of the intersubjective engagement and the emergent third is colored accordingly. Hence I offered my subjectivity to Bernard in a register that accorded with the dimension of mentalization and containment that predominated at that time in the treatment. In fact, might we not think of dimensions of intersubjectivity much like, and in accordance with, the dimensions of mentalization outlined by Lecours and Bouchard. So, for instance, when a patient, like Bernard, is immersed in the motoric mode (moving around the room, adjusting his clothes, or watching videos) one accommodates the dimension of one's subjectivity such that it *accords and harmonizes* with this dimension. One could also say that when Bernard was in evacuative mode, I companioned him by simply receiving and containing his mode as a showing, a dimension of relating, that asked to be received on its own terms. This form of intersubjective companioning offers the potential for psychic transformation, such that Bernard and I together began to elaborate what had previously been unthinkable and unavailable for experience (and evokes Trevarthen's "cooperative intersubjectivity," so crucial for ordinary mental and relational development). In a zone of "joint consciousness in companionship" we came to spontaneously elaborate and incarnate a primal experience of amniotic twinship. This coheres with Ogden's image of transference as "an act of experiencing for the first time (with the analyst and in relation to the analyst) an emotional event that occurred in infancy or childhood, but was impossible to experience at the time" (Ogden, 2012, p. 41). Here we have a clinical process that imbricates object relations theory, intersubjective engagement, and the position of the unobtrusive relational analyst.

Conclusion

I have outlined a register of relational psychoanalytic work that involves an expansion of the use of the analyst's subjectivity so as to work with patients and states that are not accessible to reflection and exploration in the verbal and related realm. The unobtrusive companioning register allows access to unformulated, non-represented, and unspeakable realms of the patient's experience and emphasizes the sometimes quiet and deeply engaged accompanying of the patient. Primacy is given to the patient's idiom, psychic signature, and illusion. The analyst is interested to embrace and accompany the patient into inner darkness, emptiness, wordlessness, and raw emotions rather than seeking to move the patient into more related and dialogic registers. The analyst harmonizes with the dimension of mentalization and subjectivity that emerges as the patient's internal world comes to fill the space of the treatment such that new dimensions of intersubjectivity, relatedness, and internal cohesion emerge. Both analyst and patient reside within the emergent and hallucinatory field of the treatment (Civitarese, 2013; Ferro, 1999, 2002) and both find and make meaning as regressed states are lived through together in "joint consciousness in companionship." In the words of Matthew Sanford, rather than striving to overcome the darkness, we embrace and companion the patient in the emergent darkness and silence and hence engage with the "fundamental" and "essential parts" of who the patient is and thus vitalize the patient's "sense of living"(Sanford, p. 128). As Bernard said "I feel I can live."

Note

1 Certainly, much of this material might also be taken to suggest an enactment of actual violent penetration. We have talked at great length about this and for Bernard it is the father's mental violation that really resonates.

References

Anzieu, D. (2010). Functions of the skin ego. In D. Birksted-Breen, S. Flanders, & A. Gibeault (Eds.), *Reading French psychoanalysis*. London and New York: Routledge.

Bach, S. (1994). *The language of perversion and the language of love*. Northvale, NJ: Aronson.

Bach, S. (2006). *Getting from here to there: Analytic love and analytic process*. Hillsdale, NJ: The Analytic Press.

Bach, S., Grossmark, C., & Kandall, E. (2014). The empty self and the perils of attachment. *Psychoanalytic Review, 101*, 321–340.

Balint, M. (1968). *The basic fault: Therapeutic aspects of regression*. New York: Bruner/Mazel.

Bass, A. (2014). Three pleas for a measure of uncertainty, reverie, and private contemplation in the chaotic, interactive, nonlinear dynamic field of interpersonal/intersubjective relational psychoanalysis. *Psychoanalytic Dialogues, 24*, 663–675.

Bion, W. R. D. (1957). Differentiation of the psychotic from the non-psychotic personalities. *The International Journal of Psychoanalysis, 38*, 266–235.

Bion, W. R. D. (1962). *Learning from experience*. London: Tavistock.

Black, M. J. (2003). Enactment: Musings on energy, language and personal growth. *Psychoanalytic Dialogues, 13*, 633–655.

Botella, S., & Botella, C. (2005). *The work of psychic figurability: Mental states without representation*. Hove, New York: Routledge.

Brazelton, T. B. (1993). *Touchpoints: Your child's emotional and behavioral development*. New York: Viking.

Civitarese, G. (2013). The inaccessible unconscious and reverie as a path of figurability. In H. Levine, G. S. Reed, & D. Scarfone (Eds.), *Unrepresented states and the construction of meaning: Clinical and theoretical contributions*. London: Karnak Books.

Cooper, S. (2014). The things we carry: Finding/creating the object and the analyst's self-reflective participation. *Psychoanalytic Dialogues, 24*, 621–636.

Corbett, K. (2014). The analyst's private space: Spontaneity, ritual, psychotherapeutic action, and self-care. *Psychoanalytic Dialogues, 24*, 637–647.

Director, L. (2009). The enlivening object. *Contemporary Psychoanalysis, 45*, 120–141.

Director, L. (2014). The object invades: Illustration and implications. *Contemporary Psychoanalysis, 50*, 437–458.

Ferenczi, S. (1928 [1955]). The elasticity of psycho-analytic technique. In S. Ferenczi, *Final contributions to the problems and methods of psycho-analysis*. New York: Basic Books.

Ferro, A. (1999). Narrations and interpretations. In A. Ferro, *Psychoanalysis as therapy and storytelling*. London: Routledge.

Ferro, A. (2002). *In the analyst's consulting room*. Hove, New York: Routledge.

Ghent, E. (1990). Masochism, submission, surrender. *Contemporary Psychoanalysis, 26*, 169–211.

Green, A. (1999). *The work of the negative*. London: Free Association Books.

Grossmark, R. (2009). The case of Pamela. *Psychoanalytic Dialogues, 19*, 22–30.

Grossmark, R. (2012a). The unobtrusive relational analyst. *Psychoanalytic Dialogues, 22*, 629–646.

Grossmark, R. (2012b). The flow of enactive engagement. *Contemporary Psychoanalysis, 48*(3), 287–300.

Harris, A. (2014). Introduction. *Psychoanalytic Dialogues, 24*, 615–620.

Klein, M. (1946). Notes on some schizoid mechanisms. *The International Journal of Psychoanalysis, 27*, 99–110.

Lecours, S., & Bouchard, M. (1997). Dimensions of mentalisation: Outlining levels of psychic transformation. *The International Journal of Psychoanalysis, 78*, 855–875.

Levine, H., Reed, G. S., & Scarfone, D. (Eds.). (2013). *Unrepresented states and the construction of meaning: Clinical and theoretical contributions*. London: Karnak Books.

McGleughlin, J. (2011). The analyst's necessary vertigo. *Psychoanalytic Dialogues, 21*, 630–642.

Mitchell, S. (1997). *Influence and autonomy in the psychoanalytic situation*. Hillsdale, NJ: The Analytic Press.

Ogden, T. H. (2012). *Creative readings: Essays on seminal analytic works*. Hove, New York: Routledge.

Reis, B. (2009). Performative and enactive features of psychoanalytic witnessing: The transference as the scene of address. *International Journal of Psychoanalysis, 90*, 1359–1372.

Reis, B. (2010). Enactive fields: An approach to interaction in the Kleinian-Bionian model. Commentary on paper by Lawrence J. Brown. *Psychoanalytic Dialogues, 20*, 695–703.

Reis, B. (2011). Zombie states: Reconsidering the relationship between life and death instincts. *Psychoanalytic Quarterly, LXXX*(2), 269–286.

Sanford, M. (2006). *Waking: A Memoir of trauma and transcendence*. New York: Rodale Books.

Seligman, S. (2014). Paying attention and feeling puzzled: The analytic mindset as an agent of therapeutic change. *Psychoanalytic Dialogues, 24*, 648–662.

Slochower, J. (1996). *Holding and psychoanalysis: A relational perspective*. Hillsdale NJ, London: The Analytic Press.

Slochower, J. (2006). *Psychoanalytic collisions*. Hillsdale, NJ: Analytic Press.

Stern, D. B. (2014). Relational psychoanalysis and the inner life: Commentary on Cooper, Corbett and Seligman. *Psychoanalytic Dialogues, 24*, 676–683.

Stern, D. N. (1993). The role of feelings for an interpersonal self. In U. Neisser (Ed.), *The perceived self: Ecological and interpersonal sources of self-knowledge* (pp. 205–215). New York: Cambridge University Press.

Stern, D. N. (2010). *Forms of vitality: Exploring dynamic experience in psychology, the arts, psychotherapy, and development*. Oxford: Oxford University Press.

Trevarthen, C. (2001). Intrinsic motives for companionship in understanding: Their origin, development, and the significance for infant mental health. *Infant Mental Health Journal, 22*(1–2), 95–131.

Tronick, E. (2001). Emotional connections and dyadic consciousness in infant-mother and patient – therapist interactions: Commentary on paper by Frank M. Lachmann. *Psychoanalytic Dialogues, 11*, 187–194.

Tronick, E. (2003). "Of course all relationships are unique": How Co-creative processes generate unique mother-infant and patient-therapist relationships and change other relationships. *Psychoanalytic Inquiry, 23*, 473–491.

Winnicott, D. W. (1945). Primitive emotional development, reprinted in D. W. Winnicott, *Through pediatrics to psycho-analysis*. New York: Basic Books, 1975.

Chapter 4

The eloquence of action

Unobtrusive psychoanalytic
companioning and the growth
of mind and self[1]

> Action is eloquence.
> —William Shakespeare, *Coriolanus* (2009, p. 159)

> Often a patient's acting out may be an attempt to assist positively the
> analysis where the mind has failed.
> —Paul Williams (1998, p. 545)

With increasing frequency, we find ourselves working with patients and
states that are not amenable to verbal and dialogic engagement. Likewise,
we have become more sensitized to the pockets of regressed functioning
that reside within many patients who possess developed psychological and
interpersonal capacities. Such patients and states are challenging for psychoanalytic work that assumes some verbal expressiveness and reflective
function in the patient. In this chapter I will outline an approach that leans
on an expansion of psychoanalytic engagement and intersubjectivity to
engage with these areas.

I believe that the generative action of psychoanalytic treatment with
these patients and states, for whom mutuality and relatedness is either
limited or disturbed, accrues when a safe and welcoming place is created in the treatment for the annunciation of and engagement with these
states and ways of being. These inchoate areas of psychological functioning announce their presence in the enacted, motoric, non-symbolized,
and sensorial realm of the treatment and can appear as behaviors, reveries, somatic sensations, and emerging narratives within and between
the analytic pair or in the bi-personal field, the enacted dimension of the
treatment.

It is the companioning and engagement with these often wordless and formless states of being that, I believe, is at the core of the generative action of psychoanalysis and brings about the inner transformations that stimulate the growth of symbolic and representational capacities, such that reflective function, mentalization, self-other differentiation, regulation of affect and state, and, ultimately, greater humanity can take fertile root. Further, it is these areas of non-represented inner darkness and limit that so often leave the patient with unbearable and enduring shame, psychic pain, and inner loneliness. I foreground the analyst's unobtrusive yet engaged companioning of the patient in the flow of enactments into non-represented and non-symbolized states, which creates an address for these dimensions of being that may not be available to a treatment that places greater store on interpretation of conflict or on the examination of analyst-patient interaction. In other words, we make ourselves available to be taken into areas and states of private shame, non-relatedness, and perverse and archaic object relating.

These are often patients who were subjected to profound, early damage or environments of neglect, so that they may contend with violent inner lives and states of turbulence or emptier inner worlds and states of isolation. Such conditions disturb or constrain relatedness such that customary modes of intersubjective engagement are not feasible. It is at this level that damage occurred and continues to reside, and it is in this register that we must work. When there has been unevenness in the maturational environment, we find a similar unevenness in adult functioning. Many such patients have developed areas of competence and even stellar functioning and relatedness that, while adaptive, can serve to obscure the aspects and areas of the self that are constrained and afflicted. Such patients and states have always presented a dilemma for psychoanalytic – and indeed all mental health – practice.

Analysts since Ferenczi have looked to a more elastic approach to work effectively in these areas. Michael Balint (1968) observed that they would seem to respond well in an environment where they can settle into a form of relatedness that is less developed than that which exists between two adults: in other words, an approach to treatment that finds a way to work in the register and dimension of psychic functioning that corresponds best with their own internal world. Central to my approach is the idea that psychoanalytic healing is most effective when the analyst can find a way to be-with and to companion the patient *within* the very registers that are most damaged and constrained. Rather than attempting to find relief by bringing the patient *out* of their inner worlds of suffering and non-symbolizable psychic pain and into the light of dialogic mutuality (the world in which we analysts are frequently most comfortable ourselves), the analyst can find a way to enter *into* the world of the patient: to enter into the darkness, confusion, and non-relatedness.

When an analyst can be unobtrusive to the narrative that emerges in the mutual flow of enactment (which may be a slow burn rather than an acute fire of enactment), the story of the patient's internal world, early object relations, and areas of non-symbolized non-relatedness emerge in the field of the treatment. The boundaries of space and time become diffuse, and what emerges is a blend of past, present, and future. Lew Aron and Galit Atlas (2015) recently noted that enactments can tell us as much about the future as about the past. In saying that the analyst unobtrusively companions the patient in this flow is not to say that the analyst effaces herself. The analyst is both present as him- or herself, yet gives prominence to and surrenders to what emerges from the patient. This may involve quiet and patient waiting with the patient, or it may involve active responses to the patient's call for engagement and felt impact.

A simple example: A young man begins to miss sessions or arrive late. On some occasions, he arrives as much as forty minutes late. He does not quite know what is going on. I take it that we are hearing from a part of his inner world that has no form or outline and has yet to find "voice" in the register of the symbolized and reflective. I find myself confused and lost, yet not afraid for him or the treatment. The treatment is capturing a call from the depths, a call that has no words or form. As this continues over months, I begin to lose track of the sessions myself and often find that I cannot remember who it is that comes at his hour. My mental calendar appears to have a hole in it where he should be. We begin to find form in this absence. Rather than finding that he has absented himself from our work, I find that I am companioning him in a formless experience of absence. He has been showing me something he could not have known, and it found presence in the transpersonal field (Foulkes, 1964, 1975) that we both constituted and were constituted by. Indeed, it turned out that he had always suffered with a pervasive sense of inexplicable separateness from others. In a family where he had always been lauded as brilliant and precocious, he had always felt alone and strangely disconnected. There had been an invisible absence buried in the overwhelming presence of excitement and adulation that had surrounded him and had passed for love and attachment. He and I and the field we constituted had told the story of that absence, a story that was not yet known to him. Bion taught that it takes two people to think; I might say that it takes two people and an emergent field to tell a story. We both participated in the emergence of this unconscious narrative. The key here is to not rush to talk about, to understand, or to make meaning out of what is going on in the treatment. It is by allowing – welcoming, really – the mutual enactment to unfold over time that we find ourselves living through states of illusion and distortion and what Ogden (2005), following Bion, called shared states of "waking dreaming" that give emotional shape and human accompaniment to the patient's unconscious inner suffering. I would argue that to have tried to discuss the situation would have pulled us out of the emergent, illusory, enacted dimension of non-engagement and into the world of dialogic engagement, the very register that does not allow access to this area. As my title proposes, there is eloquence to action and to what comes to be lived through together. This is a symbolization-in-action or an enactive representation (Lyons-Ruth, 1999).

The focus is on mutual action and motoric and sensorial communication. I do feel that psychoanalysis has been bedeviled by the idea of "acting out." This concept created a binary that separates action and communication, privileges the discursive while diminishing the language of the body and of enactment. Freud himself valued action and the somatic: He regarded his first patients' bodily symptoms as communications (Freud, 1895) and repeating as a form of remembering (Freud, 1914). Lecours and Bouchard (1997) outline different dimensions of mentalization that include the somatic and motoric. These are not *not* thinking; they are thinking *in another register*! Thinking with our bodies, with our cells, and with our engagements with others – an unconscious waking dreaming together. So when a patient talks in repetitive monosyllabic cadence about obscure details of his workplace, and the analyst feels heavy with boredom and sleep, we can take a leaf out of Winnicott's book and not regard this as *not* psychoanalysis, but look for what the patient *is* showing us. And this showing is in the register of experience, rather than through thoughts, words, or concepts. We can become receptive to a world of diminished objects and non-relatedness and surrender to another kind of reality. The generative action of such a psychoanalytic treatment derives from the experience of with-ness, from companioning the patient in their darkest and perhaps most non-related and disorganized realities. Mind, mentalization, self-other differentiation, continuity, and regulation of self are generated via "joint consciousness in companionship" (Trevarthen, 2001), via "changing with" an other (Stern et al., 1985, p. 263), and through "living the full course of an experience" together (Winnicott, 1941, p. 67) without obtrusion.

I think my work with Lloyd will illustrate some of these ideas. Lloyd was a 50-year-old white American man. Despite a successful and impressive career in international business, he described a life of sorrow and neurotic symptoms that had troubled him since childhood. His marriage of more than 20 years was a source of frustration and some confusion, as was the task of bringing up three teenage girls with whom he struggled to find connection. Every day was dominated by relentless self-blame and castigation and had been for as long as he could remember. Never at ease within himself, he suffered volatile mood swings, sudden unexplainable rushes of anxiety, and plunges into listless despondence. At times, he felt terminally lonely, isolated, and empty, despite the plethora of people who populated his world. At other times, he could feel an expansive sense of liberation, fullness, and effectiveness. He described attempts to fill himself up in different domains. Eating binges and daily masturbation to pornography felt like addictions, and about one year before his call to me, he had begun an extra-marital affair with a married woman. After much consideration in his sessions, he recognized that the affair was an attempt to fill up his inner emptiness, and about one year into our work together, with much sadness, he dissolved the relationship and re-committed to his marriage and his children. He initiated couples therapy with his wife and felt that he had to address what had not been right between them from the get-go. He told me he felt that our work was helping him gain some control in his life and within himself. He had grown up scared of his father, an angry man who could fly into physical rages. He felt that his father had chronically misread him. Where Lloyd had felt fear, the father had seen aberrant behavior and punished him accordingly. He described his mother as manically peppy and unable to respond in any real way to the father's strict regime or to Lloyd himself. He found her almost impossible to genuinely connect with. He continued to make real gains in the treatment. He opened up to his wife's and others' input regarding his relationship with his children, and there were some signs of improvement with his daughters. With great effort of will, he ceased the daily masturbation that had been a feature of his life since his early teenage years and engaged with what felt like real psychological exploration in the treatment. So far, so good!

However, alongside all of these and further developments in his treatment and life, I had the growing sense that something was not real. It was as if he were constructing the emotions: The language was too precise and insightful, too psychoanalytic in a way. So when one day he mournfully described the experience of talking in sessions as losing himself – "It's all gone, dumped out of me. But where has it gone? It's all gone" – I heard the presence of a more primitive, less developed dimension to his functioning where words and feelings are things and what passes between people are primal and concrete objects.

After about 18 months of treatment, he told me a dream that seemed to reverberate with my growing sense that there was another dimension that was not being connected with. In the dream, a journalist and a photographer were talking about an article concerning him, Lloyd, in a prominent literary magazine. "It was very important. But I couldn't get into the conversation. I was losing control of my own story. I was no longer a part of it. I could see the written article. It was very sad." We talked about how this captured the sense that he was not truly inhabiting his own life and the treatment itself: that we, our mature adult and intelligent selves, were living a version of how he felt within himself continuously; that we were talking about him as an interesting object of narration rather than truly connecting to his inner world and some form of sadness. We were losing touch with some other dimension, something that would be potentially closer to whom he might truly be. He commented that this felt inevitable and very familiar to him in all his relationships, including his wife and daughters. He knew that the masturbation, the affair, and other activities, including fights with his wife and children, had been attempts to connect to himself and to feel alive and real, but he was at a loss to say anything further about what *real* might be. Over time, he began to manifest emanations from another dimension, from the motoric and non-symbolized dimension. I first noticed this when, one day, I went to greet him in the waiting room, and he was drinking a glass of water. I gathered that he had gone into the small pantry in my office suite, had taken a glass from the cabinet above the sink, and had filled the glass with tap water. He had not asked permission and made no mention of it. I asked if he had in fact found the glass and water in the pantry, and he confirmed this and carried on with the session with no further mention of it. I registered an uncomfortable feeling and asked myself if I felt violated by this unusual crossing of the boundary that separates the public space of the waiting room and the private space of the pantry. In truth, I concluded, there was a feeling of violation, but also surprise and curiosity. After all, I did not truly mind. I recognize this kind of experience that is both real but also not quite real. I take it that this is a signal that we, the analytic dyad, are entering into another realm, a dream-space that is transitional and potentially transformative in nature, perhaps a harbinger of the "rest of him," the parts of him that were not represented in any form in his. He was showing what he could not tell. I surrendered to the flow of enactive engagement. The idea here is that to inquire further is to engage with the verbal and related dimension, represented in the dream by the conversation between the journalist and the photographer, the very dimension from which we were trying to free ourselves. I needed to companion him in this new register and wait unknowingly to see what would emerge, sensing that this may be the path to a shared symbolization-in-action of his pain.

Further communications in this motoric and non-symbolized register followed. More water was drunk, plates taken on which to put his morning muffin, and the kettle used to boil water for tea. I kept in mind the idea that the motoric and sensory modes are not to be regarded as *not* mentalized, but *are* mentalizations in another dimension, another language. Subsequently, he came to a number of sessions in a manifestly altered state. He seemed totally deflated and bereft of any energy. All he could do was mumble that he could not speak or do anything. These sessions were terribly trying for me. I sat with him and initially tried to engage him but did not persist. He simply did not and, I gathered, could not respond. He was truly lifeless. He could not describe these states more than to say that they sometimes came upon him. There is no time here to tell you details about how things progressed. Suffice to say that he continued to communicate in this domain, moving chairs around the office, asking me to sit in different alignments with him, which I did, ultimately settling on an arrangement that could not have been closer: his chair immediately in front of mine so that we could register each other's breathing. My sense at this time was that he was desperate to impact me, to experience me as alive, and that this needed to happen in the direct motoric and concrete realm. More than simply feeling intruded upon, I felt drawn into a world where desperation and intrusion were the only pathways to shared life. Then his mother appeared in a dream. She seemed totally lifeless. He described how his mother's body in the dream recalled for him a dead body he had once seen as a young man. He focused on the visceral registration of a body without life in it. We talked about the deadness he had always carried and the sense that inside his mother's peppy exterior was a barren death-like wasteland. Soon after this, he met with his mother and they had a meaningful conversation unlike any they had had before, during which she described being deeply depressed and unable to cope emotionally when he was a child. Lloyd considered that in fact she did and continues to love him but has been constricted in her ability to do so, particularly in those crucial early years. "I have been so dead inside all this time," he said. "So I use self-attack, masturbation, and sex to feel located." I said, "Yes: to feel yourself and alive." He seemed visibly moved and paused for a while, seeming to breathe and take this in. He then turned away annulling the connection: "So what? What difference does all this make?" He looked at me, as if challenging me to not let him get away with it. We had developed a way of being together that demanded full honesty on both our parts, as best we could. So I said, with a sense of real pain: "Oh no! You just turned away. You made the aliveness dead." And he pushed: "Yes, but how does it feel to *you*?" "Well," I said, sensing that nothing short of emotional honesty would do, "it actually leaves me feeling ashamed for having felt well-connected to you just then." "That," he said, "is very helpful." He paused and hung his head for a long while. He finally said sorrowfully: "All my life I have been ashamed." His whole mood and presence seemed more alive, real, and connected – and deeply sad. We had lived through a companioned experience together.

We had lived a narrative that not only gave shape to the unbearable shame at having an internalized no-life mother, an absence of life-generating energy, but also fertilized the very inner capacity to symbolize what had previously been unrepresentable. In the language of Bion (1967), the beta dimension of motoric impulse had been transformed by a companioned experience into a felt experience of shame. The meaning of his motoric actions was not *revealed* but was *established* together (Killingmo, 1989). His behavior was in no way an attack on the analytic relationship or even simply intrusive. Rather, it was an eloquent signal of the emergence of an area that until then had had no affective shape or substance. It was a progressive attempt to integrate areas of undifferentiated affects and states of psychological disaster into the safe space of our work. It was Winnicott (1974) who suggested that some patients require a breakdown in the treatment, and by companioning him in this regressed area, in the motoric register, the pathway to thought and emotional realization was opened. This small vignette illustrates that my work with Lloyd was not aimed at getting him somewhere else, to an area of verbal or cognitive reflection or to greater mutual recognition. Rather, we proceeded in the register of companioning. It is this register, I suggest, that generated a path to effectance (White, 1959), agency (Rustin, 1997; Sander, 2008), and to ownership of his own analysis and consequently of his own mind, affect, and experience.

Note

1 Paper presented at the 2017 National Institute for the Psychotherapies Annual Conference, "The Generative Action of Psychoanalysis," New York City, February 2017.

References

Aron, L., & Atlas, G. (2015). Generative enactment: Memories from the future. *Psychoanalytic Dialogues, 25*, 309–324.

Balint, M. (1968). *The basic fault: Therapeutic aspects of regression*. New York: Bruner/Mazel.

Bion, W. R. (1967). A theory of thinking. In *Second thoughts: Selected thoughts on psychoanalysis*. Northvale, NJ: Jason Aronson.

Foulkes, S. H. (1964). *Therapeutic group analysis*. London: Karnac Books.

Foulkes, S. H. (1975). *Group analytic psychotherapy: Method and principles*. London: Karnac Books.

Freud, S. (1895). The psychotherapy of hysteria. In J. Strachey (Ed. & Trans.), *The standard edition of the complete psychological works of Sigmund Freud* (Vol. 2, pp. 253–305). London: Hogarth Press.

Freud, S. (1914). Remembering, repeating and working through. In J. Strachey (Ed. & Trans.), *The standard edition of the complete psychological works of Sigmund Freud* (Vol. 12, pp. 145–156). London: Hogarth Press.

Killingmo, B. (1989). Conflict and deficit: Implications for technique. *International Journal of Psychoanalysis, 70*, 65–79.

Lecours, S., & Bouchard, M. (1997). Dimensions of mentalisation: Outlining levels of psychic transformation. *International Journal of Psychoanalysis, 78*, 855–875.

Lyons-Ruth, K. (1999). The two-person unconscious: Intersubjective dialogue, enactive relational representation and the emergence of new forms of relational representation. *Psychoanalytic Inquiry, 19*, 576–617.

Ogden, T. H. (2005). On holding, containing, being and dreaming. In T. H. Ogden, *This art of psychoanalysis: Dreaming undreamt dreams and interrupted cries* (pp. 93–108). London: Routledge.

Rustin, J. (1997). Infancy, agency and intersubjectivity. *Psychoanalytic Dialogues, 7*, 43–62.

Sander, L. (2008). Thinking differently: Principles of process in living systems and the specificity of being known. In G. Amadei & I. Bianchi (Eds.), *Living systems, evolving consciousness, and the emerging person: A selection of papers from the life work of Louis Sander* (pp. 215–233). New York: The Analytic Press.

Shakespeare, W. (2009). *Coriolanus*, III, 2, 95, Folger Shakespeare Library, p. 159.

Stern, D., Hofer, L., Haft, W., & Dore, J. (1985). Affect attunement: The sharing of feeling states between mother and infant by means of intermodal fluency. In T. Field & N. Fox (Eds.), *Social perception in Infants*. Norwood, NJ: Ablex.

Trevarthen, C. (2001). Intrinsic motives for companionship in understanding: Their origin, development, and the significance for infant mental health. *Infant Mental Health Journal, 22*, 95–131.

White, R. (1959). Motivation reconsidered: The concept of effectance. *Psychological Review, 66*, 297–323.

Williams, P. (1998). Reply to commentaries. *Psychoanalytic Dialogues, 8*(4), 531–546.

Winnicott, D. W. (1941 [1958]). The observation of infants in a set situation. In D. W. Winnicott, *Through pediatrics to psychoanalysis: Collected papers* (pp. 52–69). New York: Basic Books.

Winnicott, D. W. (1974). Fear of breakdown. *International Review of Psychoanalysis, 1*, 103–107.

Chapter 5

Enactment

The total situation

> We are all talkers
> It is true, but underneath the talk lies
> The moving and not wanting to be moved, the loose
> Meaning, untidy and simple like a threshing floor.
> —John Ashbery, "Soonest Mended" (1997, p. 232)

Introduction

In this chapter, I will propose that alongside enactments of trauma and early object relations, we might consider a register of the incarnation of Total Situations, outlined by Melanie Klein and later applied to the transference by Betty Joseph, in the treatment dyad and field. I will suggest that Klein's concept of total situations invites a vector of understanding of analytic process and enactments that can bring the patient's internal world and unrepresented states to life in the field of the treatment. In particular, I will propose that Klein's concept of total situations asks the analyst to appreciate and welcome the totalistic nature of the patient's experience.

Unlike Klein and Joseph, whose clinical methodology preceded the contemporary focus on intersubjectivity, enactments, and field theory, I argue that both patient and analyst participate in the incarnation and living through of these total situations, and that when allowed to unfold by an unobtrusive relational analyst, the field of the treatment itself can embody, incarnate, and bring to life these non-represented and unformulated total situations. In doing so, I emphasize areas of functioning that are not mentalized or symbolized and are most commonly found in the dimensions of somatic, motor activity (Lecours & Bouchard, 1997) and the transpersonal field. The focus of this register of psychoanalytic engagement is the analyst's companioning of the patient within these states (Grossmark, 2016) as a means of fostering the growth of inner psychic capacities, rather than interventions oriented to bringing the patient into areas of greater ego strength or psychological development. An explication of Klein's concept of Total Situations will be followed by a close reading of Betty Joseph's (1985) seminal paper "Transference: The Total Situation." I will highlight the clinical wisdom that I draw from this paper and contrast her clinical methodology to that of a more contemporary unobtrusive relational analyst, where there is value placed on the psychoanalytic companioning of the patient into regressed and non-represented states (Grossmark, 2012a, 2012b, 2016).

Total situations

During the famous "controversial discussions" in the British Psychoanalytical Society between 1941 and 1945, Melanie Klein outlined the infant's progression from the paranoid-schizoid position to the beginnings of the depressive position and suggested that "the infant goes through a series of total situations in the first year of life" (King & Steiner, 1991, p. 839). The hallmarks of the depressive position are the development of whole objects and the sense of loss, mourning, and ambivalence that are contrasted to the split and fragmented objects that characterize the earlier months dominated by the paranoid-schizoid position. With the onset of depressive position functioning, there is a gradual integration of experience, and the infant is able to relate to the mother as a whole object and draw together his or her own experience in a more consistent and coherent manner. Thus, self and other begin to develop. However, these developments – as always, in Kleinian theory – come at a price. Now able to conceive of the object as separate and whole, the infant grieves the malignant consequences of his or her own destructive impulses. The idealized mother of earlier infancy loses its extreme goodness and badness. There is gradual integration and the mother is now increasingly seen as flawed and imperfect rather than idealized. This compounds a sense of loss and melancholy, hence Klein's naming this the "depressive position." Out of this storm of painful experiences can come such crucial developments as a sense of guilt, morality, integration, concern, and the wish for reparation. Likierman (2001) points out that it is when outlining the depressive position that Klein seems to reach for and describe the infant's actual experience more than at any other place in her writings, and it is in describing the volatile mix of these experiences – whether flooded by guilt, filled up with hope, or paralyzed by overwhelming anxiety – that Klein suggests that at each moment, the infant is experiencing a total situation. As the infant slaloms back and forth from more integrated and whole experiences to more fragmented, primitive functioning, there is a continual immersion in "complete" or total situations. Likierman puts it succinctly: "Klein was increasingly convinced that within the infant's most primitive framework each part of the ambivalent relationship is a total situation that overwhelms him in turn" (p. 122).

Furthermore, in reaching for a way to delineate the experience of internal objects, Likierman sees Klein as suggesting that the infant does not experience internal objects as such, so much as total situations comprising an all-engulfing experience that is fundamentally in the realm of primary sensations and the somatic. These are pre-verbal, non-represented, and unformulated experiences that are a ubiquitous part of normal development, rather than specifically the consequence of non-recognition, neglect, or trauma.

It seems that this rendition of total situations obviates the need to locate the experience as either in the individual or between individuals: It is a totality, a surround. I will return to this notion later and discuss the implications for the analyst when working in the realm of total situations that can come to "overwhelm" the treatment. Indeed, Klein (1952) herself some years later drew on the notion of total situations to outline her understanding of the transference. Emphasizing her view that every detail of the clinical encounter is regarded as a manifestation of the transference, she wrote: "It is my experience that in unraveling the details of the transference it is essential to think in terms of *total situations* transferred from the past onto the present, as well as of emotions, defences and object relations" (p. 437, emphasis in original).

Always focused on the manifestations of the earliest relations to the primal object, primarily the mother/breast, Klein (1952) suggests that regardless of the patient's reports of current and daily life, we do well to maintain our focus on the nature of the object relationship in the transference:

> for the patient is bound to deal with conflicts and anxieties re-experienced towards the analyst by the same methods he used in the past. That is to say, he turns away from the analyst as he attempted to turn away

from his primal objects; he tries to split the relations to him, keeping him either as a good or as a bad figure: he deflects some of the feelings and attitudes experienced towards the analyst on to other people in his current life and this is part of "acting out."

(p. 437)

Years later, Betty Joseph elaborated upon these evocative ideas, and in her landmark paper, "Transference: The Total Situation" (1985), she outlined a conception of transference as a dynamic and constantly moving situation, "a framework, in which something is always going on, where there is always movement and activity" (p. 156). She emphasized that the transference relationship reveals not only relationships with early objects, but also the internal world of the patient and how that internal world is responding to the ongoing analytic relationship; all material, including "such things as reports about everyday life, and so on, gave a clue to the unconscious anxieties stirred up in the transference situation" (p. 156). The treatment relationship can therefore be viewed as a manifestation of total situations. Hence, there is a broad focus on "everything that the patient brings into the relationship" (p. 157). The analyst is to focus on "what is going on within the relationship" and to constantly consider how the patient is "using the analyst alongside what he is saying" (p. 157). The focus of psychoanalytic understanding is therefore shifted from the interpretation of the content of the patient's words in terms of their unconscious meaning to a more all-encompassing registration of the ongoing relationship that the patient is unconsciously creating in the analytic situation. This relationship manifests the internal world of the patient, the patient's objects relations and internal structure. In other words, patients do not *tell us* about these aspects of their internal world so much as *show us* in the way that they relate to and use the analytic situation and the analyst.

In tuning one's analytic ear to this register of unconscious communication, the analyst must use his or her countertransference, which is, according to Joseph (1985), the "essential tool of the analytic process" (p. 157). In a remarkably contemporary formulation, Joseph notes that the analyst must focus on how patients "convey aspects of their inner world built up from infancy – elaborated in childhood and adulthood, *experiences often beyond the use of words*, which we can often only capture through the feelings aroused in us, through our countertransference" (p. 157, italics added). She exhorts us to focus on this level, and to not become solely captured by the manifest material of the patient's verbal reports. In doing so, she tilts into another prescient formulation, implicitly referring to the personality as comprised of multiple "parts": "If we work only with the part that is verbalized, we do not really take into account the object relationship being acted out in the transference" (p. 158).

The implication, familiar to readers of the contemporary relational literature, is that the personality is comprised of a multiplicity, and much as I have argued in this volume and elsewhere (Grossmark, 2012a, 2012b, 2016), she suggests that when the primary focus is on the verbalized and formulated parts, or states, of the personality, the analysis may exclude less organized and non-represented memories, states, and areas of non-relatedness. In other words, the manifestation of early total situations may be obscured by the engagement with the patient's more verbal, organized, and related states. Such a sensibility seems to harmonize with the contemporary interest in what is non-represented (Levine et al., 2013) and unformulated (D. B. Stern, 1997, 2010 and the overall thrust of this book. Joseph (1985) emphasizes this again and introduces the idea that there is a living out of the patient's early forms of relatedness and, I would add, non-relatedness:

> Interpretations dealing only with the individual associations would touch only the more adult part of the personality, whereas the part that is really needing to be understood is communicated through the pressures brought to bear on the analyst. We can sense here the living out in the transference of something of the nature of the patient's early object relationships, her defensive organization and her method of communicating her whole conflict.
>
> (p. 159)

Joseph illustrates these ideas of transference as "basically living, experiencing and shifting – as movement" (p. 160) with some clinical examples. The red thread that runs through the examples is that the analyst must attend to the object relationship developing in the transference and hold off on interpreting the manifest material. The analyst can observe the deeper and more fundamental conflict and total situation that is afflicting the patient as it is experienced in the analytic relationship.

In one of Joseph's examples, we see a frustrated supervision group struggle to find coherent meaning in the case material presented, despite "sensitive," "adequate," and insightful comments and interpretations from the presenting analyst and seminar members. Gradually, it dawned on the seminar members that their lived experience of confusion and dissatisfaction in the seminar was itself a narration of the patient's internal world, the core to the transference and the case itself. They were experiencing "the patient's inner world in which, the patient, could not understand, and more, could not make sense of what was going on" (p. 158). Moreover, "she was demonstrating what it felt like to have a mother who could not tune into the child and, we suspected, could not make sense of the child's feelings either, but behaved as if she could, as we, the seminar, were doing" (p. 158). In other words, the seminar was living out the total situation of the patient's internal world and experience as a child.

Another case illustrates how a patient's conflicts and destructive, triumphant, locked-in, and internally trapped self came to be lived out in the treatment as he, the patient, did not allow himself to be helped by Joseph, and induces in the treatment the total situation of the very claustrophobic trapped inner world that prevents any open engagement with life and others. I will examine this case in detail shortly.

Transference: the total situation and psychoanalytic technique

Before expanding on the value that I find in the notion of total situations as outlined by Klein and Joseph, I would like to take a moment to describe Joseph's technique and to consider how a conceptualization of *enactments* of the total situation may afford a wider range of clinical possibilities than her concept of *transference*: the total situation. Such a reading honors her contribution while underlining the potential value in the current embrace of intersubjectivity and enactments, and in particular, the concept of the flow of enactive engagement (Grossmark, 2012b).

Despite her descriptions of psychoanalytic treatment as dynamic and constantly in motion and her foregrounding of the realm of the non-verbalized parts of the personality that are inevitably "lived out" in the treatment, I imagine that Betty's Joseph's clinical technique as described in this and other papers (e.g., Joseph, 1985) might strike many contemporary analysts as overly reliant on interpretive technique. Furthermore, as I mentioned above, she wrote before the notions of intersubjectivity, mutuality, and enactment became staples of much contemporary understanding of clinical process. Hence she conceives of herself as outside of the clinical interaction and possessed of a clear and unimpeded understanding of that process.

One example might capture this. After a period of sustained improvement in his life, the locked-in young male patient mentioned above complained to Joseph that she had not given sufficient attention to a ritual he had developed while extremely lonely at boarding school. He would

> take a tin, or a cardboard box, and cover it extremely carefully with canvas. Then he would dig out the pages of a book and hide his cigarette box inside the cover. He would then go into the countryside alone, sit, for example, behind an elder bush and smoke: this was the beginning of his smoking. He was lonely. It was very vivid. He subsequently added that there seemed to be no real pleasure in the cigarettes.
>
> (p. 162)

In a complex interpretation – the richness of which I cannot capture in this brief sketch – Joseph "showed" him how he was trapping her and that he was struggling to give up his excitement at triumphing over his elders (remember, he would hide behind an elder bush) and to give up "some of the pleasure in defeating me" (as he continued to smoke despite gaining no pleasure) (p. 162). The reader has little doubt as to the accuracy of Joseph's interpretation on one level, but the patient's response is telling: He "tended to agree" with Joseph but went back to the cigarette box and expressed sadness and resentment that she had not given this story the attention that it deserved. Where a contemporary analyst, whose focus includes the intersubjective matrix of the field, might take the patient's critical comments as commentaries on the field, and hence be open to examining (and perhaps even sharing) some of his or her own process in an attempt to understand the patient's experience of the analyst here, Joseph resorts to interpreting and she places the whole situation within the patient rather than in the dyad itself. Insisting on her original interpretation that he was resisting the experience of goodness, she "also showed him his resentment at the fact that his feelings had shifted, he had lost the uncomfortable blocked mood" (p. 162). The patient agrees but continues (rather pluckily, I think) to press upon Joseph that she left the story of the cigarette box too quickly. Joseph continues to interpret, suggesting that he is scared of her seducing him out of his safe negativity and withdrawal and that he is scared of experiencing excited and warm feelings toward her. She does not appear to me to be wrong when she comments on the struggle to free the patient from his masochistic orientation to life. However, Joseph does not consider that it might in fact be true that she was seducing the patient into more positive feelings for unconscious reasons of her own, and that she actually didn't give sufficient attention and credence to the story of the cigarette box, as the patient persists in telling her. She may, in fact, have gone too fast.

Rather than purely seeing this sequence as transference and projection, we might view this today as an enacted narration of the patient's relationship with his mother or of his internal life. We might hypothesize that the mother herself sought to focus on and seduce him into the positive, rather than staying with the hurt and vulnerable states that he found so lonely. Hence we have an enactment of the very loneliness he is describing. Or we might see this, much as Joseph does, as a rendition of the patient's internal struggle with a deep inner loneliness and isolation; perhaps she is embodying the internal saboteur (Fairbairn, 1952) that attacks any vulnerability and neediness with the push for greater insight and suppression of the scared and lonely child within. Whether or not these are accurate considerations, by conceptualizing this kind of interaction as a mutual enactment rather than a one-directional transference, we are open to both considering the subjectivity of the analyst *and* the patient as well as continuing the focus on the way that the patient's internal world is gripping and shaping the field of the treatment as it unfolds: creating a total situation that involves the subjectivity of the analyst as well as that of the patient. Such a formulation is, in fact, closer to Joseph's understanding of the supervision group mentioned before, where she suggests that the whole group participated in an unconscious rendition of the patient's internal world.

I would also highlight Joseph's emphasis on showing the patient how he is resisting the potential value of the work they have done. From my perspective, Joseph is embodying an approach common to many psychoanalytic and psychological treatments: the will to move the patient *out* of their suffering and misery, to bring them *out* of the total situation that is emerging in the treatment. From my perspective, the psychoanalytic setting offers a unique opportunity to enter *into* and companion the patient *within* the total situation of the world they psychically live within. Rather than seeking to move the patient *out* of this world, as Joseph seems determined to do with her patient, I would be more inclined to be unobtrusive to the patient's desire to have the analyst be with him as he dwells in the treatment, *within* this terribly alone and locked-in world. The patient seems to be crying out for more recognition of this isolated part of him. I would be interested to allow myself to surrender to the flow of this enactive engagement and to be taken by him behind the elder bush and into the yet-to-be articulated experience of being buried in a tin within a book behind a bush.

Psychoanalytic incarnation of total situations

This critique of Betty Joseph's clinical praxis need not obscure the great value in her elaboration of Klein's conception of transference as a total situation, and I will argue that there is real clinical profit in conceptualizing enactments as total situations. Accordingly, we can conceptualize enactments as the living out of these experiential total situations that involve "aspects of (the patient's) inner world built up from infancy . . . experiences often beyond the use of words" (Joseph, 1985, p. 157), such that what was not represented due to either ongoing developmental trauma, non-recognition, or neglect can find form and incarnation in the treatment. These enactments are total in that they involve the patient, the analyst, and the field of the treatment in an evolving hermeneutic process of narration and transformation.

The "experiences beyond the use of words" have remained in the domain of the non-represented and yearn for an "other," a container, to metabolize, alphabetize, and give life to these total situations. From the neo-Bionian perspective, this process is primarily driven by the analyst's reverie and careful verbalization of the understanding of the field that develops between the patient and analyst (Ferro & Civitarese, 2015). From the relational perspective, there is emphasis on the use of the analyst's own experience to articulate the emergence of dissociated self-states. The analyst may engage the patient in a consideration of what might be happening in the treatment, such that what has been dissociated can come to be felt, experienced, and engaged with as lived experience.

Borrowing from both these perspectives, I would suggest that the analyst orient his or her attention to the emergence of total situations in the treatment. Such total situations involve the analyst, the patient, and the field of the treatment (rather like Betty Joseph's supervision group). The patient and analyst both comprise the total situation, like the field, and live within it. This is why it can be difficult to grasp what is unfolding until one catches on to the particularities of the specific analytic relationship one finds oneself living within. The total situation becomes incarnated in the treatment. I choose this word because of the physical and somatic implication. Both the analyst's and the patient's bodies, minds and spirits, if you will, are engaged. Furthermore, *incarnation* seems to capture the other-worldly, both the here-and-now as well as the from-some-other-time-and-place sense that these situations evoke for both patient and analyst. They are the incarnation of what is not purely in the realm of lived experience or reality: It is the emergence of inner worlds of illusion where fragmentation, fantasy, the imaginary, and the liminal preside.

The analyst can be unobtrusive yet deeply engaged with this process of incarnation and can expect to live within these total situations in altered, strange, and disturbing psychic spaces together with the patient. The task is to flow with this process and not to impede it with precipitant interpretations or inquiry, to not ask the patient to step into a more developed self-state that is more available for verbal description and is more oriented to what the analyst may regard as reality. Quite the opposite: The analyst is to companion the patient into these worlds of experience and pre-experience where objects may be bizarre, split, or barely discernible and where reality may take a back seat, if it is present at all. The naming, alphabetizing, or understanding comes not from the realm of the verbal (although, ultimately there will be words). It comes from joining and companioning the patient in this liminal world of illusion where the verbal is yet to set foot. Such lonely and unarticulated landscapes are best "understood" by the experience of being companioned in the very same register: the non-verbal. The emphasis is on this register of being-with the patient. In this endeavor, I join other contemporary psychoanalytic writers who seek to describe different dimensions of being-with patients and who place complex notions of a psychoanalytic being-with at the core of psychoanalytic healing (Eshel, 2013; Reis, 2009, 2010, 2016). This way of knowing and understanding the patient is fluid and dynamic and shares much with the how the Boston Change Process Study Group (Nahum, 2008 and Lyons-Ruth 1998) have described implicit relational knowing that coheres and grows in the treatment interaction itself.

There is an evocation here of Ogden's (2005) perspective when describing Bion's thoughts about "waking dreaming" that analytic work must provide a setting in which the conscious can become unconscious rather than making the unconscious conscious via interpretation or premature understanding. Verbal "understanding" comes later, but few would disagree that that understanding can at best only approximate the experience itself. That liminal world can only be known via a lived experience, and it is the analyst's task to avail him- or herself of that experience, of that total situation.

I would also echo Klein's observation that the experience of total situations is "overwhelming" to the infant (Likierman, 2001, p. 122). The overwhelming nature of the clinical experience when one is involved in the enactment of early total situations is often deeply disturbing to the analyst and the patient and can be experienced as a threat to the integrity of the treatment. It is the very overwhelming quality of the analyst's experience or countertransference that signals the emergence of a total situation in the treatment. By its nature, a total situation involves the predominance of a split, sometimes concrete, primal and non-reflective *total* experience.

Much treatment relies upon the multiplicity of the patient (Bromberg, 1996, 2000, 2006). We need the verbal, mature, and reflective patient to work with us as we attempt to alphabetize and make meaning out of the material. But the notion of the total situation asks us to consider the mutual regression to these all-encompassing situations where there is no other place to stand, at least for the moment; where paranoid-schizoid dynamics are a *totality*; where the analyst really is a part object; where the world is concrete; where the multiplicity of alternate self-states is not available; where intersubjectivity is but a distant echo; and where doer/done-to dynamics, paranoia, projection, and non-object-relatedness can dominate. The immersion in the "PS" (paranoid-schizoid) experience is a totality in itself, and the lubricating and creative work of "PS< >D" (shifts between the paranoid-schizoid and depressive positions) is not available. In the idiom of Bromberg's (1996) dissociation theory, rather than "standing in the spaces," we accommodate to a world where there simply is no space to stand. The suggestion here is that the work of transformation and psychic integration comes not from flight from these paranoid-schizoid total situations but from an embrace, acceptance, and companioning *within* these dark spaces. The analyst does not flee from them, and the treatment can maintain its integrity in the face of them: Both analyst and patient survive them.

The incarnation of total situations echoes the early Kleinian emphasis on understanding these shared clinical experiences as the living out of the patient's early and ongoing *internal worlds* and *imaginary* registers, the world of the patient's illusion. Recall Melanie Klein's view that the infant does not experience internal objects as such, so much as total situations comprising an all-engulfing experience. This is distinguished from the contemporary notion of enactment as a re-enactment of dissociated trauma, where trauma is seen as that which happened but is yet to become experienced and owned as part of the self and that which resides in dissociated self-states, or not me (Bromberg, 1996, 2000, 2006; D. B. Stern, 1997, 2010, 2015). The suggestion here is not to replace this conception of the enactment of early trauma, but to introduce another register that is often present that also involves the patient and the analyst, best captured by the notion of incarnation of total situations.

Incarnation of total situations in the field of treatment

It is hard to think about the incarnation of total situations without recalling the work of Ferro, Civitarese, and other neo-Bionian field theorists, particularly those that emphasize the oneiric dimension of psychoanalysis.

In brief, from this perspective, the field is comprised of the conscious and unconscious realms of both analysand and analyst. In every analytic relationship, both participants develop powerful unconscious fantasies of the nature of the dyad as it unfolds and the nature of the cure that is wished for and feared. At any given moment, the analyst can understand what is happening in the treatment according to the current state of fantasies about the relationship. These ideas have been adapted and expanded by many contemporary writers, most notably Ferro (1999, 2002, 2009) and Civitarese (2012, 2013), who provide numerous examples of how they understand the treatment process in terms of a constant message from the unconscious of the dyad regarding the state of the relationship. The rather decentering idea here is that the message comes from the field, rather than from either participant. The field, constituted by both participants' conscious and unconscious fantasies and fears, their worlds of internal object relations, and the transferences that ensue, develops and takes on a transformative and generative quality of its own. Narratives and worlds are generated that are more than the sum of their parts (i.e., the internal and intersubjective worlds of the patient and analyst).

From my perspective, I regard the analyst's surrender to the unfolding of emergent meanings in the flow of enactive engagement as the creation of the space within which the field itself can flow and find meaning. As the analyst and patient both take this "hermeneutic ride" together, the field is allowed to unobtrusively express itself. *The analyst is unobtrusive to the unfolding of the field.* The field affords the emergence of unformulated and non-represented meanings that cannot be articulated in language, but are *lived through* together (Joseph, 1985) and find form in this companioned experience.

The field can be said to incarnate the total situations of the patient's internal world. From this perspective, it is not only a matter of considering the unconscious worlds of both analysand and analyst, but to think about the emergence of the field, a surround that captures and embodies the total situation. The field can be regarded as a total situation itself, and when the analyst can allow the field to take shape and grow, the total situation can become manifest and can be lived in together with the patient. Such an experience can be disturbing and disorienting to the analyst because of the predominance of bizarre and hallucinatory phenomena, and as mentioned above, because of the overwhelming quality of the paranoid-schizoid dimension of experience. However, it is my contention that the accompanying of patients in this kind of total situation can promote a transformative experience for the patient.

Taking Betty Joseph's lead, I will illustrate these ideas with two examples, one from an individual psychoanalysis and one from a group situation.

Phoebe

Phoebe's mother never let her breathe her own breath, never let her think her own thoughts or feel her own feelings. "She was always all over me," Phoebe cried as she lay on the couch. "And now I can't feel my own body: I don't know whose body this is." Phoebe's mother had pressed Phoebe so close to her, driven by fears of trauma and the terrors of an alien world in a new country. Most confusing to Phoebe was the suffocating quality of her mother's idealizing love. Phoebe, the only child, was at the very center of her mother's life. Everything she did was wonderful and exceptional, her body the pinnacle of beauty, her thoughts the effusions of genius, her athletic abilities Olympic feats. Phoebe grew up feeling totally loved. She recalls running home from school to just be surrounded by her mother's presence. "I'd run down the street to our house, my heart pounding, feeling that there was not a happier kid in the world." However, when asked to separate, by going to camp or sleepovers with relatives, Phoebe found herself paralyzed by panic and nameless terrors. Relationships in school were fraught with missteps, faux pas, and social blindness. The world was bemusing, and she secretly felt unprepared, clumsy, and somehow separated from her peers. Home was everything. She knew she was angry with her parents for isolating her in their tiny universe. "I was not prepared to leave paradise: How could they have left me naked in the world?"

Her intellect, wit, and personal charm carried her through college and into eventual marriage and motherhood. Now as a senior executive in an insurance company with a devoted husband, young grandchildren, and a flourishing family, she has come to treatment because of a lingering sense of emptiness and almost constant panic. She mentions in passing in the initial consultation that she has never loved anyone. I ask her what she meant and she pauses, confused. "Did I say that? Well . . . my mother loved me, but." And the story unfolds. She does acknowledge the love her husband and grown children feel for her, but wonders if it is real. It has the quality of a movie she watches, rather than an emotional reality that she lives and inhabits. She does love her family, she says, but it doesn't feel entirely real. She wonders and worries about one son's apparent alcoholism and her daughter's husband's coldness and resentment. She cries alone in the bathroom at work, pleading with her mother to let her be. Her mother has been dead for over ten years. In the treatment, we travel back in time; the smells, sounds, and atmospheres of her family home fill the room. Small and vivid memories are alive and present: a cold, angry response from her mother when she talked of being disappointed that she didn't make the field hockey team, or professed to uncertain struggles with her homework. It is with pain, wonder, and liberation that she begins to spell out what she has always thought but never articulated: Her mother needed her to be perfect and had very little sense of, or even interest in, who she might be as her own person. A slight cough would elicit manic medical examinations of her body from her mother, cold and hot compresses applied, doctors called and general panic in the household. Phoebe cries as she exclaims: "She didn't have any interest in *me*!"

Treatment proceeds well, and Phoebe compares our work favorably with previous therapy experiences. She addresses her son's drinking and begins a conversation with her daughter about her marriage. People comment that she seems to be feeling better these days. I feel comfortable and helpful with Phoebe. She seems to listen intently to what I say and to value our work. She makes notes after sessions and often brings the notebook in to read me further thoughts she has jotted down in between sessions. An atmosphere of mutual idealization buoyed our work.

As might be expected, the dynamics of Phoebe's relationship with her mother began to infuse the treatment. Beyond any consideration of particular moments in the sessions, a total situation of mutual suffocation began to emerge in the enacted dimension of the treatment. Phoebe found herself panicking as vacations approached, and once on a vacation she cried alone in the bedroom, weeping and hugging herself, crying out "I am so alone. I have no one. Not my mother, not my husband, not Dr. Grossmark, no one." She reproached me on her return: "You weren't there when I needed you."

One of her sessions is scheduled after my lunch break. I return to the office one day to find her sitting outside the office suite, weeping. I am ten minutes early for the session. She says that she knows the time but was paralyzed with panic: "He [Grossmark] has left me, he doesn't care about me; it's all about him." Her rage with me for abandoning her intensifies. She lies on the couch and imagines me reading or dozing behind her. Yes, this is transference: She is experiencing me much as she experienced her narcissistic mother. She knows this. I think it is fair to say that this is a version of what Joseph would call a total situation transference that colors every moment of the treatment: her behavior in the session, her thoughts, fantasies, dreams, and sensations both in and related to the treatment. What is also compelling to me, however, is that these dynamics are not solely in the province of her transference, of her mind alone. They are also emerging in the field of the treatment. You see, the truth is that at this point, in a way, I *was* abandoning her. I found myself increasingly suffocated by her and by the whole situation. What had first appeared as a very rewarding engagement in the treatment – her notes, her dreams, her insights – now came to feel like demand and suffocation. I did not look forward to her sessions; in fact I rather dreaded them and I struggled with all manner of distractions while she talked. It was indeed hard to stay with her. Hence the Total Situation was not solely in the transference but was an ongoing enacted register in the treatment in which we were both involved, unconsciously and ineluctably.

I felt drawn into a very particular world where we were both trapped and trapping of each other. Perhaps this was an enacted rendition of Phoebe's early relationship with her mother, where her mother, bringing her own narcissistic vulnerabilities, found herself as trapped and erased by her infant's high-drive demands (Ellman, 2010; Pine, 1985) as the young Phoebe was by her mother: certainly the incarnation of Joseph's (1985) description of "aspects of their inner world built up from infancy – elaborated in childhood and adulthood, *experiences often beyond the use of words*" (p. 157, italics added). The field of the treatment was saturated in this dynamic. For a period of time, there was simply nowhere else to stand for either of us.

Rather than interpret, I companioned her in this ever more claustrophobic and unsettling landscape. "It is so very hard when it feels like I have abandoned you," I would aver. "Yes," she would agree, "it is terrifying." And then the entombing panic: "But at my age: Why all of this? How come I am not over this? Why so much suffering?" I would experience a gentle kind of asphyxiation. The unspoken horror began to announce its most unwelcome appearance in mutual enactment: She was deeply identified with her mother and was staunchly protective of that identification.

This formulation is not far from Joseph's understanding of her young male patient I mentioned earlier, who described his ritual of the cigarette box. Joseph construed this as transference and saw interpretation of the total situation as the only possible intervention. My feeling, repeated throughout this volume, is that unobtrusively companioning the patient within the emerging enactment of the total situation and living it with the patient in the present, provides the intimate recognition and knowing of the patient that lays the foundation upon which reflective function and coherent emotional experience can grow.

Thus, Phoebe dreamed that she was on an airplane flight from Europe. The seat was too small, and there was not enough legroom. She had to squirm to try to get comfortable. The more she squirmed, the more her movement seemed to draw the surround around her and pack her in. Ultimately, she could not move at all and abandoned herself to the feeling of being totally constrained. She saw a drawing – an outline, really – of herself in a tight little box.

Many angles on the dream were examined. Certainly, she was immediately aware that the dream captured the constraints of her mother's mind and her mother's needs. The airplane journey to Europe evoked her parents' migrations, her attempts to move away from them, and the overall terrifying feeling that the more she tried to define her own space and growth, the more she was trapped and almost strangled in her mother's mind. The rudimentary outline drawing of her captured a sense that there was little left of her own substance, more an empty outline where there should have been a living, breathing human. Most troubling to her was the strange sensation of comfort and surrender as the constraint became tighter. She suggested that it captured a suffocating version of swaddling; it is soothing even as it constricts. "Indeed," I reverberated, "in a strange way, it has been comfortable and safe, just like it used to be at home." She agreed, and we considered that the constriction and impingement was as much her own creation as her mother's, a manifestation of a paralyzing identification. She was scared by the thought and spoke it with fear: "Oh no, I am just like her! I guess there was no choice."

Picking up the "no choice," we talked about the inevitability of this kind of dynamic and its ubiquity in her life. It seems to always be happening. Someone is always being impinged upon or impinging, disappointing or disappointed. Her inner experience was similarly contoured. In a private, unformulated register, she had always lived in the Total Situation of her early relationship with her mother's mind, and it infused "everything that the patient brings into the relationship" (Joseph, 1985, p. 157).

I would suggest that being companioned and recognized in the emerging enactment of this suffocating and total dynamic fertilized the seeds that would become the dream. Once able to dream, the field shifted. We could talk about and look at that image of her, scrunched up and coiled in her own suffering and safety. She began to see herself and her inner need to hold on to her own mother via her distorting internalization. For the first time, she talked about a low level of resentment and anger that seemed to hover in every relationship in her work and with the family. She was, it turned out, as intolerant and impatient with others' independent minds as her mother had been of hers. She agreed and was intrigued to think through with me the ways that our relationship seemed to capture this very dynamic too. Rather than isolating the dynamic within her mind alone, we could look at how we had been living this very situation over and over, and I could offer resonant pieces of my own experience of feeling trapped with nowhere else to stand. She found these sessions useful and even exciting and felt free for the first time to consider that she had been holding on to her mother all of this time. And so gradually her depression and anger have transformed into mourning and grief. Her inner life is beginning to make sense to her.

Enactment: the total situation in a group analysis

In Betty Joseph's first example of transference, the total situation was of a supervision group that ultimately realized that their lost and confused experience when talking about a patient captured the patient's internal world. I would like to briefly mention an example of the enactment of a total situation in a group analysis. This clinical material is mentioned in much greater detail in Chapter 9 and illustrates how the whole group can come to enact and live through the non-symbolized total situations of the group members' early years.

In short, the group struggled with Gregory, who was dismissive and haughty toward the other group members and the whole endeavor. His repetitive complaint, wrapped in contempt for the group, was that no one in the group really understood him or was helpful to him. This aroused ire in other group members, who felt that he had consumed a good amount of group time talking about his abusive upbringing, and that they had offered their care and forbearance. The group became deeply frustrated with Gregory, who threatened to leave amidst a torrent of recriminations. Only when I noticed that he seemed lost and confused during one session did it become clear to me that we – Gregory, the group-as-a-whole (the field), and I – had all been engaged in living out the total situation of chronic and damaging misattunement that had completely dominated his development and now characterized his inner and relational world. I mention this example to complement the case of Phoebe and to illustrate once again how the total situation arises not only in the transference, but in the mutually enacted dimension of the field of the treatment involving both patient and analyst, and in this example, the group-as-a-whole as well.

Conclusion

In this chapter, I have suggested that there is much utility in Melanie Klein's concept of total situations and Betty Joseph's elaboration of transference as a total situation. I have furthered this elaboration to include enactments in the field of treatment and have suggested that an unobtrusive yet present and engaged analyst can facilitate the emergence of total situations in the treatment that include the analytic dyad and group. By allowing the total situations to unfold and fill out the field, and by going further *into* these enactments of total situations rather than trying to bring the patient and oneself *out* of them, the analysis (or group analysis) can become the address where the pain can finally be companioned and suffered, so that the patient's internal and relational world can come to have meaning and movement rather than static emptiness and isolation.

References

Ashbery, J. (1997). *The mooring of starting out: The first five books of poetry.* Hopewell, NJ: Ecco Press.

Bromberg, P. M. (1996). *Standing in the spaces: Essays on clinical process, trauma and dissociation.* Hillsdale, NJ: The Analytic Press.

Bromberg, P. M. (2000). Potholes on the royal road: Or is it an abyss? In *Awakening the dreamer: Clinical journeys* (pp. 85–107). Mahwah, NJ: The Analytic Press.

Bromberg, P. M. (2006). *Awakening the dreamer: Clinical journeys.* Mahwah, NJ: The Analytic Press.

Civitarese, G. (2012). *The violence of emotions: Bion and post-Bionian psychoanalysis.* London: Routledge.

Civitarese, G. (2013). The inaccessible unconscious and reverie as a path of figurability. In H. Levine, G. S. Reed, & D. Scarfone (Eds.), *Unrepresented states and the construction of meaning: Clinical and theoretical contributions* (pp. 220–339). London: Karnac Books.

Ellman, S. (2010). *When theories touch: A historical and theoretical integration of psychoanalytic thought.* London: Karnac Books.

Eshel, O. (2013). Patient-analyst "withness": On analytic "presencing," passion and compassion in states of breakdown despair and deadness. *Psychoanalytic Quarterly, 132*(4), 925–963.

Fairbairn, W. R. D. (1952 [1994]). Endopsychic structure considered in terms of object relationships. In W. R. D. Fairbairn, *Psychoanalytic studies of the personality* (pp. 82–136). London: Tavistock Publications.

Ferro, A. (1999). *The bi-personal field: Experiences in child analysis.* London: Routledge.

Ferro, A. (2002). *In the analyst's consulting room.* London: Routledge.

Ferro, A. (2009). Transformations in dreaming and characters in the psychoanalytic field. *International Journal of Psychoanalysis, 90,* 209–230.

Ferro, A., & Civitarese, G. (2015). *The analytic field and its transformations.* London: Karnac Books.

Grossmark, R. (2012a). The unobtrusive relational analyst. *Psychoanalytic Dialogues, 22,* 629–646.

Grossmark, R. (2012b). The flow of enactive engagement. *Contemporary Psychoanalysis, 48,* 287–300.

Grossmark, R. (2016). Psychoanalytic companioning. *Psychoanalytic Dialogues, 26,* 698–712.

Joseph, B. (1985). Transference: The total situation. In M. Feldman & E. B. Spillius (Eds.), *Psychic equilibrium and psychic change: Selected papers of Betty Joseph* (pp. 156–167). London: Routledge.

Katz, G. (2014). *The play within the play: The enacted dimension of psychoanalytic process.* London, New York: Routledge Taylor & Francis Group.

King, P., & Steiner, R. (Eds.) (1991). *The Freud-Klein controversies, 1941–1945* (pp. 823–843). London: Routledge.

Klein, M. (1952). The origins of transference. *International Journal of Psychoanalysis, 33,* 433–438.

Lecours, S., & Bouchard, M. (1997). Dimensions of mentalisation: Outlining levels of psychic transformation. *International Journal of Psychoanalysis, 78,* 855–875.

Levine, H. B., Reed, G. S., & Scarfone, D. (Eds.). (2013). *Unrepresented states and the construction of meaning: Clinical and theoretical contributions.* London: Karnac Books.

Likierman, M. (2001). *Melanie Klein: Her life in context.* London: Continuum Press.

Lyons-Ruth, K. (1998). Implicit relational knowing: Its role in development and psychoanalytic treatment. *Infant Mental Health Journal, 19,* 282–291.

Nahum, J. P. (2008). Forms of relational meaning: Issues in the relations between the implicit and reflective-verbal domain: Boston change process study group. *Psychoanalytic Dialogues, 18*(2), 125–148.

Ogden, T. (2005). On holding containing, being and dreaming. In T. Ogden, *This art of psychoanalysis: Dreaming undreamt dreams and interrupted cries* (pp. 93–108). London: Routledge.

Pine, F. (1985). *Developmental theory and clinical process.* New Haven, CT: Yale University Press.

Reis, B. (2009b). Performative and enactive features of psychoanalytic witnessing: The transference as the scene of address. *International Journal of Psychoanalysis, 90,* 1359–1372.

Reis, B. (2010). A human family: Commentary on paper by Elisabeth Fivaz-Depeursinge, Chloe Lavanchy-Scaiola, and Nicolas Favez. *Psychoanalytic Dialogues, 20*(2), 151–157.

Reis, B. (2016). Monsters, dreams and madness: Commentary on 'The Arms of the Chimeras'. *International Journal of Psychoanalysis, 97,* 479–488.

Stern, D. B. (1997). *Unformulated experience: From dissociation to imagination in psychoanalysis.* Hillsdale, NJ: The Analytic Press.

Stern, D. B. (2010). *Partners in thought: Working with unformulated experience, dissociation and enactment.* New York: Routledge.

Stern, D. B. (2015). *Relational freedom: Emergent properties of the interpersonal field.* London: Routledge.

Chapter 6

Everything happens at once

The emergence of symmetric enactment[1]

> Deep in the forest there's an unexpected clearing which can be reached only by someone who has lost his way.
> —Tomas Transtromer, "The Clearing" (1987, p. 139)

> The only reason for time is so that everything doesn't happen at once.
> —Albert Einstein (Oz & Oz-Salzberger, 2012, p. 108)

Introduction

When unobtrusively companioning the patient in the flow of enactive engagement, the analyst finds him- or herself entering altered states of consciousness as the treatment space and field come to capture the unconscious inner object world and idiom of the patient. These states may be momentary and fleeting and take the form of brief hallucinatory images, reveries, or dreams, or they may be durable states that are evoked and lived within over long periods of analytic work. One might say that the analyst comes to live within the unconscious of the patient. Such states arrive in the realm of the sensory, tactile, and the non-represented sense of things and can involve brief or prolonged disturbances in the sense of reality, time, and space. Working this way has opened up some unique and moving journeys with my patients, as I have tried to convey in the foregoing chapters in my work with Kyle (Chapter 1), Reuben (Chapter 2), Bernard (Chapter 3), and Lloyd (Chapter 4). Their everyday experiences of themselves, others, and the world were shaped by the early failures of the maturational environment such that the basic structures of experience – time, space, and differentiations between people and things and between self and others – were distorted, muted, or at least vulnerable to disruption. This chapter discusses enactments of disruptions in temporal and spatial reality.

Bion (1967) has suggested that the dichotomy of unconscious and conscious is akin to that between infinitude and the finite and that consciousness is "won from the dark and formless infinite" (p. 165). Thus, in each of the treatments I have described, it can be said that I came to companion the patients in the realms of the dark and formless infinite where time and space dissolved and were sometimes reconfigured such that linearity, the separations between past, present, and future, before and after, and inside and outside were diffused or vanished altogether. These shared experiences kindled a deep sense of intimacy and trust in the treatment and seem to have been central to the psychoanalytic healing that took root. In what follows, I will elaborate on the dimensions of timelessness and spacelessness that can emerge when the analyst is unobtrusive to the flow of enactive engagement with patients for whom time and space are collapsed and transfigured. It is a transcendent encounter when one finds oneself outside of time, in Einstein's words, in the realm where everything happens at once

I will begin with some thoughts about our relationship to linear time and its alternatives and then engage with Riccardo Lombardi's (2016) embellishments of Ignacio Matte Blanco's (1975, 1988) theory of the unrepressed unconscious and its relation to states of timelessness and spacelessness. While drawing much wisdom from this theoretical perspective, I will distinguish my clinical approach from that of Lombardi. As will become clear, Lombardi seeks to create clinical healing via the introduction of time, boundary, and limit into the clinical process to draw the patient out of the states of timelessness and boundarilessness. I will contrast this with my clinical approach and will offer a clinical vignette to illustrate the value of unobtrusively companioning patients within this dimension.

Time and timelessness

Many from Freud onwards have contemplated the curious, compelling, and somewhat mind-bending experiences of time in psychoanalysis. But few have so profoundly drawn our attention to the organizing qualities of time than Einstein in the epigraph to this chapter. I do not read Einstein as suggesting a socially constructed idea of time, but rather a consideration of the function of time itself. And by suggesting that time's function is to organize "everything" in sequence – or else everything would happen all at once – he opens the possibility that there are realms of existence, not simply experience, that are located and locatable outside of the linear concept of time, an idea that coheres with Bion's (1967) conception that finitude (time) is won from a primordial zone of timelessness.

In their fascinating essay "Time and Timelessness," Amos Oz and Fania Oz-Salzberger (2012) review the multiple conceptions of time that inhere in biblical, ancient, and mystical Jewish experience. They suggest that our modern, post-Enlightenment linearity – where "time's arrow" (Amis, 1991) moves ineluctably forward, forever "progressing toward a glorious future, or rushing toward a dismal man-made catastrophe" according to a "secular linearity . . . and leading to a future instigated by us" (Oz & Oz-Salzberger, 2012, p. 109) – is but one conception of a barely graspable phenomenon. Ecclesiastes' sentiment that "that which hath been is that which shall be and that which hath been done is that which shall be done" (p. 109) not only suggests a circularity rather than a linearity, but also uncannily points to what we now commonly encounter in our psychoanalytic practice in the form of enactments and trauma.

Oz and Oz-Salzberger note that in the Hebrew language one stands with one's back to the future, facing the past: "The Hebrew word *kedem* means 'ancient times' but the derivative *kadima* means 'frontward' or 'forward'. The Hebrew speaker," they conclude, "literally looks frontward to the past" (p. 118): an ancient rendition of *Nachträglichkeit*.

In these considerations and evocations of the biblical and archaeological past, we paradoxically find the deconstruction of the ultimate binary – the future and the past. I find such thinking liberating and very relevant to the kinds of clinical engagements I am addressing here, where the flow of enactive engagement reveals a zone where future and past are not strung together on the filament of linear time. Entering such states with these patients can evoke a profound sense of being lost, but rather than see this as an impediment to the psychoanalytic process, I lean on the sentiment of the poet Tomas Transtromer (1987), quoted above, and regard the process of being lost together as the very pathway itself to the "unexpected clearing" (p. 139) where unbidden healing and realization can arise (D. B. Stern, 1997).

Bi-logic, symmetry, and asymmetry

Without time, everything would happen at once, says Einstein, and in so doing he introduces the specter of a reality where infinity and non-differentiation predominate, a world of non-contradiction and non-distinction between objects, selves, and time. It so happens that this is the very world of Freud's unconscious (Freud, 1900, 1915) familiar to us from our dreams and nightmares and central to the theory of the unrepressed unconscious developed by the Chilean psychoanalyst Ignacio Matte Blanco (1975, 1988).[2] If we are to unobtrusively allow the unconscious process of the patient to fill the treatment space, we can anticipate living within a realty that is shaped by these very characteristics.

Matte Blanco echoes Freud's suggestion that alongside the repressed, dynamic unconscious, we find the unrepressed unconscious whose signature is timelessness, spacelessness, and sameness. Unlike the repressed unconscious where organized memories and thoughts are pushed out of consciousness via repression, in the unrepressed unconscious we encounter an altered state where there is no separateness, no contradictions, or distinctions – only the stuff of dreams: condensation, negation, displacement, and above all, "the replacement of external by internal reality" (Lombardi, 2016, p. 4). There are no beginnings and endings, only infinity. The unrepressed unconscious is subject to the laws of symmetrical logic or the "principle of symmetry" (Matte Blanco, 1988, pp. 43–69) according to which elements are symmetrical with – the same as – other elements. The hallmark of the principle of symmetry is the dissolution of time, space, and categories: Everything is the same. By virtue of these features, there is no cognizable thought or at least process that we would recognize as organized thought. There is no "inner" and no "outer" and hence no "self" and "not self" (Rayner & Tuckett, 1988, p. 37) and no differentiation between self and other. This is the inner world of the "basic matrix" (Matte Blanco, 1988, pp. 193–195).[3] In such an experiential world, not only does everything happen at once, but everything is the same, a "formless infinity" (Lombardi, 2016). So, for example, one might find that a patient experiences all elderly men just as he experienced his grandfather, or all movement, whether walking or airplane flight, is experienced as being dropped or disintegrating. There is no distinctness, only a general equivalence between people, things, and the elements of life. Patients do not describe this internal state of affairs. Rather, this "formless infinity" is encountered via non-differentiated sensations and diffuse mental presences.

While this may seem to be far from our everyday experience and perhaps purely in the domain of psychosis – a patient I worked with in the inpatient unit in the State Psychiatric Hospital experienced every sentient being as a monster about to attack her, and every inanimate object as a sharp knife – we need only search our own dreams to find evidence of this blurring of categories or observe the equivalences that underlie day-to-day phenomena of transference and distortion in our patients to see versions of this phenomenon.

This logic of symmetry is paired, in Matte Blanco's schema, with asymmetrical logic, which we would recognize as ordinary logic, the basis of cognition and thinking. Here we see the presence of differentiated categories that are stable across time, finiteness, and separateness. There is sequence and order such that thoughts can take shape and be linked to other thoughts.

We all live with an admixture of these two logics – symmetrical and asymmetrical. This is the "bi-logical system." The human mind is comprised of this "bi-logical system," and there is a constant flow of bi-logic, the blend of the infinite and finiteness, that allows for the many layers of our human experience (Matte Blanco, 1988, pp. 184–200).[4] Hence we all have access to states of infinity and oceanic sensations – such as when we are in love, in the throes of intense passion or hate, or swept up in beautiful and moving music. We also have the capacity for empathy and attunement that contain elements of symmetry: We can feel for another due to the degree that we can experience some quality of sameness. And we also live in a world where it is an unremarked given that we adhere to asymmetrical logic where there are boundaries and differentiations between things and experiences. Hence we can think and proceed with organized thought in a world where time moves sequentially, and one can rely upon the consistency of things and their substance and thus experience effectance (White, 1959) and agency.[5]

Symmetric enactment

I have found Matte Blanco's work and Lombardi's elaboration of symmetry and asymmetrical logic illuminating when working with the patients and states I am addressing in this volume. I unobtrusively companion these patients into and through mutual regressions where the inner world of unconscious process comes to dominate the treatment, where boundaries between self and other blur, and where time and space dissolve: when everything happens at once. In such diffuse mental spaces, I have found it orienting to think that I am joining them in the internal spaces of their minds where symmetry is powerfully present, where asymmetrical logic is greatly reduced, and where the structure of experience and relatedness is altered. I come to understand from inside the enactment what it is like to live in their inner, non-conscious worlds where reality and time are distorted and fluid, where self and other are not distinguished. Such patients primarily communicate in the dimension of sensation and the motoric, and much of the treatment and enactment emerges in the realm of mutual impact and action. These are states and happenings that do not lend themselves to verbal and related inquiry. They ask for a different form of psychoanalytic engagement. Surrendering to the mutual flow of enactive engagement, I am able to companion these patients in the register of symmetry – timelessness, spacelessness, and non-differentiation – without the disturbance of interpretation or analysis. The emphasis is on being-with (Reis, 2009) the patient in these states in a companioned and implicit register. Such a being-with endorses the core self that is wrapped in the diffusion of the primitive states. It is this unobtrusive being-with – living with and being deeply affected – that is healing and that fertilizes the growth of asymmetrical logic, the elaboration of mind, and the alphabetizing of experience in and of itself.

I refer to this shared experience as "symmetric enactment." Both patient and analyst come to live in the world of timelessness and spacelessness where bodily sensations and action predominate. Thus, we can say that the analyst is unobtrusive to the emergence of symmetric enactment. When companioned in this world that has been sequestered in private inner spaces, the patient is no longer alone with this private madness (Green, 1986) and can begin to integrate their own bi-logic world so that they can utilize their access to the world of symmetry in a fuller and more reality-oriented – asymmetrical – existence. They can move to a place where everything happens at once *and* one thing follows another.

Lombardi, bi-logic, and clinical technique

I will now take a close look at how Lombardi approaches clinical work with these states and will outline some thoughts about how such states can arise, not simply within the patient, but within the enacted dimension of the treatment (Katz, 2014) involving both patient, analyst, and the field in a world of timelessness and spacelessness in symmetric enactment. I will suggest that the unobtrusive relational analyst can companion the patient in the flow of enactment of these experiences, and it is this accompaniment that fosters the spontaneous emergence of separateness, distinction, containment, and external reality – "the clothing for thought" (Lombardi, 2016, p. 27).

But first, I will take a closer look at some of Lombardi's descriptions of his clinical work with these states in order to contrast it with the work of the unobtrusive relational analyst. Lombardi's approach seems to exemplify a traditional psychoanalytic orientation that seeks to move the patient out of areas of regression – in this case, areas of symmetric immersion. The analyst is situated outside the fray and can introduce the voice of reality, time, and space. Lombardi's approach with regressed patients is to gradually introduce what he calls finitization and asymmetry. By this, he means boundaries, limit, and time, such that the qualities that will afford the outline of experience and thought can grow in the treatment. There is much focus on the body and somatic sensations as it is through such somatic awareness that finitization and asymmetry take root, which is to say that it is through the experience and awareness of our bodies as they function, grow, and change that we come to recognize boundary, time, and finiteness.

Lombardi (2016) recognizes that in these areas where self and other are indistinct, transference interpretations will be of limited use, and thus he is studious to avoid interpreting the transference. He writes:

> It should be noted that, from a technical point of view, at this depth of mental functioning a psychoanalytic approach based on systematic transference interpretation is counterproductive to the extent that in the deep unconscious, characterized by the emergence of somatic sensations (Freud, 1940), the distinction between external and internal vanishes and the analyst finds himself functioning essentially as the analysand's counterpart, i.e. as a sort of imaginary twin (Bion, 1950) who contributes significantly to the functions of containment and asymmetrization of the sensory-emotional experience that the analysand is going through.
>
> (Lombardi, 2016). (p. 22)

In other words, when patients are dominated by states of symmetric logic and the treatment is pervaded by a symmetric transference – where there is no self and other, no inside and outside, and no sequential, linear time – the analyst finds him- or herself in a profound participation within the process, acting as if s/he were the patient's imaginary twin or "counterpart." Such language would appear to resonate deeply with the concepts of the unobtrusive relational analyst, who surrenders to the flow of enactive engagement and companions the patient into the depths of their inner worlds. Indeed, Lombardi (2016) evokes a "somatic countertransference" (p. 125), where "the deepest levels of the process of analytic elaboration engage his or her psychophysical subjectivity to a profound and pervasive extent" (p. 125), and "the totality of the analyst's person is involved" (p. 124). Certainly, these are sentiments that would seem to fit very kindly with the ethos of this volume.

Lombardi's clinical position avoids giving transference interpretations precisely because he finds that the analyst is engaged in a profound participation and at-one-ment with the patient. However, he limits his interventions almost exclusively to interpretations that describe the patient's world and mental processes to the patient as he sees them from his perch outside of this profound participation, and he offers a running commentary on these processes and dynamics.

For instance, he describes his work with Giorgia, a woman in her forties (Lombardi, 2016, pp. 163–165). Giorgia spent the initial period of the treatment lying on the couch and frequently moving around the room. She told Lombardi that this was because she "goes backward and forward in time" (p. 163). Lombardi understands that this is an expression of the lack of temporal boundaries.[6] Subsequently, the patient enters a session and states: "The difficulty of talking here is that it does not continue. I have made many mistakes: I cannot start all over again" (p. 163).

Lombardi writes that he was scared by the intense self-attack he experienced in Giorgia and understood that her perception of temporality – the beginning of the session – evoked a sensation of guilt and persecutory self-attack. He tried to calm her, saying, "You interpret everything as your mistakes, as your fault, even the breaks between a session and the next. To end and to start new experiences, however, is necessary in life" (p. 163). His aim is to help Giorgia with the confusion and persecutory aspect of temporality, to bring her into a more comfortable sense of shared temporality, and to lessen a sense of guilt that she seems to have whenever anything ends. Hence he offered the observation that ending and beginning things is part of life and growth. Giorgia is quiet for a while and then says, "It's my birthday today: forty-five years ago I was born and I screamed. Perhaps I must scream here too" (p. 164).

Lombardi responds to the concreteness of her response and says that he places himself "on her wavelength" (p. 164) while attempting to introduce greater symbolic functioning. He says, "By suggesting you should scream, you acknowledge your hatred and your suffering are ways of feeling that you have been born and that you are now alive" (p. 164).

Lombardi tells us that he is on Giorgia's wavelength, but his interventions are designed to put a distance between Giorgia and that very wavelength. His statements would seem to ask Giorgia to step out of her current state and to reflect upon her own functioning along with such abstract considerations as the necessity of beginnings and endings as a part of life. I understand that placing this distance is a part of Lombardi's intention: to gradually introduce elements of asymmetric logic, time, and space. But we might ask if there is another way of engaging Giorgia that might also accrue such elements yet not ask her to distance herself from her own sensations and to abandon a self-state where reflective functioning and linearity are much reduced.

I would suggest that unobtrusive companioning of Giorgia in these states might offer her a way to settle into her own wavelength held in the lap of the mind of the analyst (Alvarez, 1992). For instance, when she began by saying that "the difficulty here is that it does not continue," could one join her and say, "It is so hard when things cannot be relied upon to simply continue" and allow her to know that she is understood and not alone?

When she talks of screaming in response to her forty-fifth birthday, we might recognize that a birthday is a marker of the passage of time, and that for Giorgia this brings terrible pain. Winnicott suggested that the mother's introduction of time to the infant constitutes the infant's first experience of an external reality that is not governed by the infant's own internal rhythms and sensations and is therefore the first experience of separation and loss of omnipotence. We can assume that when Giorgia was an infant, she was not helped to manage these experiences by a containing mother's mind. So when she experiences the passage of time on her birthday and wants to scream, can we not say that she is once again crying out for a containing mind to help her deal with the pain of separation and loss of omnipotence? As a child, we can imagine, she was left alone with the resulting disorganizing primal anger and hate, and these became lodged inside her as internalized persecutory objects. One wonders if Lombardi's insistence on talking from outside of her experience is an enactment of this very early abandonment and her scream is a manifestation of this primal frustration that she turns on herself as self-hatred. Recall that Lombardi felt "almost paralyzed and frightened by the persecutory atmosphere Giorgia activates against herself" (p. 163). We cannot know what this may manifest, but the kind of thought that I would consider is whether we are internally witnessing/living out a scene where a mother/analyst is terrified by her own infant's mind and emotions. A mother who is terrified of her infant's mind in this way would be most prone to not being able to join with the child's reality. Lombardi's paralysis and fear would seem to me to be a powerful communication in the enacted dimension of this treatment.

The session with Giorgia continues. Giorgia tells Lombardi that she did not take her watch with her when she went out of town. Lombardi tells her that when she leaves the session she throws away her internal clock and her capacity to think so as to not experience the boundaries of the session. Giorgia agrees and tells Lombardi that she recognizes that "one starts again even if one stops." Lombardi, sensing the growing integration within the patient, tells her that she is "always the same, in the past as in the present. It is this that allows you to have continuity, to end today's session and to come back for tomorrow's" (p. 165). The session ends with Lombardi aware of Giorgia's greater connection to herself and to him, and he tells us that, movingly, their eyes met on her way out.

Among the striking and engaging features of this clinical process is the analytic progression from Giorgia's disorganized functioning and avoidance of temporality to her engagement with time and object- and self-continuity, which seem to enhance self-other recognition. But we also notice that Lombardi is always talking about Giorgia to Giorgia, in keeping with an analytic stance wherein the analyst views the internal workings of the patient's mind from outside of the interaction and can tell the patient about this with surety and authority. There are no questions or reflections, no mirroring or resonance, and no consideration that Giorgia and Lombardi might be participating in an emergent field, even if that field is dominated by symmetrical logic and diffusion. Lombardi does not regard Giorgia's wish to scream as a call to be companioned in her symmetric state where time and differentiation are unbearable. Rather, Lombardi's approach is to bring her out of that state. Such an approach – which is ubiquitous in much clinical work – asks Giorgia to abandon her inner reality and to work with Lombardi in the territory that he – like most analysts – is most comfortable in: that of asymmetrical logic where time and space are coherent and where thinking and verbal understanding is paramount. However, as I have described, it would seem that the attempt to move Giorgia out of her symmetric state is itself an enactment: where Lombardi plays the role of a mother who cannot join the child where the child is and consistently seeks to have the child relate to her on her (the mother's) terms. If we hypothesize that the relationship between Giorgia and her mother was afflicted by such a dynamic, it might explain some of her symptomatology. When a child is not known for who she is and cannot feel consistently held in the mother's mind, time, space, and continuity of self and other are interrupted and damaged. Hence we might understand Giorgia's struggles with constancy and temporality as a manifestation of not being held or welcomed in her mother's mind. Accordingly, we might see her scream as a call to Lombardi to offer some recognition that she is well located in *his* mind as who she feels herself to be, and that *he* will appear when the time comes for the next session. She seeks to find continuity of self and time through knowing that she is known for who she is by her analyst and that he holds her in mind.

Thus, when Giorgia says: "Well you seem to say that one starts again even if one stops!" might one say: "Yes, and we will be here tomorrow"? I would argue that such a comment is unobtrusive in that it speaks from within her struggle and her concern about constancy and also allows the analyst to be present and not distanced from Giorgia. It attempts to join the patient in her psychic reality rather than trying to make her step outside of that reality. Above all, it says "I am with you and will continue to be here with you in this place of terror," and does not seek to draw her out of it so much as make it tolerable and therefore thinkable *on her own terms*. It does not ask her to reflect upon her own mental struggle – or the mind of the analyst – so much as respond in her own concrete register to the plea for continuity. Perhaps this plea for continuity is what is conveyed by Giorgia when their eyes meet at the end of the session. Hence we can say that where Lombardi (2016) sees "symmetrical transference" (p. 123), I would see a call from the patient for a companion in a flow of "symmetric enactment" that involves both participants.

If the analyst can be unobtrusive to the flow of this mutual enactment where, I am suggesting, Giorgia's early maturational environment and its failures is becoming a lived reality between analyst and patient in the treatment, then what had been unthought, unrepresented, and lost in time-lessness and spacelessness comes to have form in the lived experience of the analysis. This is the eloquence of action. Psychoanalytic healing then comes not from understanding from a voice outside of the patient's lived reality, but from a shared living through of the yet-to-be-thought story of the patient's early trauma. Such enactment contains not only the shape of the maturational failure and pain but also the seeds of the future, the "new beginning" (Balint, 1968) that confers the confluence of symmetric and asymmetric logic.

Mike

My work with Mike will hopefully illustrate how one might unobtrusively companion a patient in the flow of symmetric enactment and the result-ing spontaneous arising of mutual containment, asymmetry, and greater elaboration of mind.

Mike enters the office after missing Friday and Monday's sessions with-out warning or contact. It is Wednesday. He lies on the couch.

"I am so sorry I missed Wednesday's session. I wanted to come. I guess I missed Monday too. Sorry."

I am aware that my head is swimming somewhat. He clearly is out of time and does not know which day it is and which sessions he believes he has missed. I do not seek to correct him or clarify that today is, in fact, Wednesday, and that he had missed Friday and Monday, but choose to wait and see what will emerge. I align my self and my mind to this emerging symmetric reality.

Mike sighs and seems to get comfortable on the couch. "I had a dream last night. Oh but I can't remember it. Can you remember it?"

I find myself in a dreamlike zone where he believes, as if it is the most ordinary thing in the world, that I can know his dream without him tell-ing it to me. I can feel how sincerely he wishes that I recall his yet to be remembered dream. I say, "I wish I could remember it." He says, "I know. Thanks."

We are slipping into a symmetric enactment: There is little differentia-tion between his mind and mine, and temporal chronological sequence is simply not a relevancy at this point. My response is spoken from within the symmetric enactment where I find it normal and expectable that we become unclear as to what day it is and that he would assume that I know his dream even as he forgets it. I do not seek to comment upon or describe his mental process. This would require me to stand outside of the enacted zone and remove myself and him from the symmetric field that we seem to be occupying. His comment that he knows that I would like to be able to remember his dream and his "thanks" suggested to me that he understood that he was in an altered state and that he appreciated that I accepted and valued it and him without qualification, that I was right there with him and for him.

Often disoriented and confused, Mike had managed to sustain his self and his life with intermittent freelance design work that enabled him to adhere to a vague sense of impending deadlines, but allowed him to wander through his days in this timeless and diffuse manner. Mike came to see me after his girlfriend threatened to leave him due to his flatness of mood as well as his general difficulty getting anything done or showing up to anything on time. Mike was resentful about her request but desperate to sustain the relationship, and decided that he would come for treatment.

To be very brief, his early years were characterized by much inconsistency and abandonment. He was brought up by counterculture, peripatetic parents who spent much time traveling and improvising homes before moving on. He and his siblings would frequently be unsure as to their whereabouts and were often left with people they did not know while their parents completed odd jobs and various types of seasonal agricultural employment. Mike's memories of his parents are primarily sensual and dominated by the smell of marijuana, which to this day can evoke nausea and repulsion in him. Along with the terrors of often being lost and in some degree of physical danger with unknown strangers, there was the psychic damage of being forgotten about literally and emotionally by his parents. He recalls waiting, seemingly endlessly, for them to reappear. He does not know where and with whom he is in the memories, just the overpowering sense of waiting for them while hope slowly fades. His mother would be affectionate and lively – and, I gathered over time, quite manic – with the children but did not seem to hesitate before leaving them when work or some other distraction called. The family attempted to home-school the children, and it was not until they settled into one location during his first year of middle school that he could finally have a room, shared with two other siblings, a bed, a daily recognizable routine, and friendships.

When Mike came to see me, he was deeply depressed and angry. Often disoriented, he would sometimes wander around the city in a haze and become disoriented. He was taken to the psychiatric emergency room on one occasion because he had wandered into traffic and seemed oblivious. This, together with his flat mood, had pushed the girlfriend to insist that he seek psychological treatment in addition to the psychopharmacological treatment that he began following his visit to the psychiatric emergency room.

Mike is often disconnected from his own mind and body and is one of those patients who shows up in the deepest freeze of winter in a t-shirt, shorts, and flip-flops. He feels no pain or cold. So, rather than seeing my task as oriented to moving him out of his states dominated by symmetric logic and diffusion, I heard his inner scream that called me to know him in these areas and companion him there. By the time of the clinical moment described above we had worked together for over two years, and he had relaxed into utilizing the treatment to float in these spaces and to include me in them. He was coming to himself via this shared consciousness that pervaded the sessions. He became increasingly clued in to my mood and would often comment on my emotional state on entering his sessions, mostly with reasonable accuracy. I understood that he would come to life and to a greater degree of internal organization via my mind and my states rather than his own. He would use the symmetrical dimension of our fusion to his benefit.[7]

In the early spring, there are often days when the temperature outside rises to pleasantly warm levels. Hence the heat in the building where my office is located is turned off, responding thermostatically to the outside temperature. However, because the office receives little direct morning sunlight, the temperature within the office can remain quite chilly, and there is no heat from the building to warm it up. Deceived by the balmy spring air on arising that morning, I forgot about the weather conditions that can prevail in my office, and I had dressed in summer-weight clothes. By the time Mike arrived for his session some hours into my day, I was thoroughly chilled and in some discomfort. I found myself silently shivering during his session. Mike, lying on the couch, but as always aware of my bodily state, turns around to look at me. "You're cold." He sits up and gathers the warm wool blanked draped on the back of the couch, steps over to me, and drapes it on my legs. "There, that's better," he says. I find myself surprised by my own self-neglect that is now staring me in the face, along with my gratitude to Mike for being so caring. I find that his gentle caretaking words and the blanket itself warm me deeply: not simply because I am physically warmer now and am able to arrest the shivering that had gripped me, but I am also warmed emotionally. He has spoken to an old need within me to be taken care of and recognized. When faced with challenge, adversity, and downright pain, my modus operandi for much of my life had been to dig in and grimly get through without complaint. An archaic need had been awoken in me, and Mike had not simply sensed this but had responded with care. I knew that I was cold, but it had never occurred to me to take the blanket draped on the couch to warm myself. The blanket is for my patients, not for me.[8]

We could say that I was deeply involved in a "somatic countertransference" (Lombardi, 2016, p. 125). I was identified and merged with Mike, forgetting my own self and my thermostatic needs as he was wont to do when he would be hopelessly under-dressed in the winter. Perhaps I was experiencing the kind of alone and silent suffering that were so common for him in his early years, unaware that I was waiting to be found in that loneliness. Perhaps I was the mother/father unable to take care of myself and in need of a resilient parentified child who would recognize that limitation and take care of me. Perhaps all of the above, and perhaps much more. Suffice to say that I was filled with what Matte Blanco would term "sensation-emotion" (Lombardi, 2016, p. 27), and Mike was on that very wavelength such that he could respond in kind. We were living together in this world of symmetric sensation-emotion. His action not only clothed me and soothed my physical suffering, but clothed these inchoate sensations in thought. Thus, I felt that Mike and I together had created the enactive conditions within which his early, lonely suffering could be tended to in the present via his caring for my shivering and my old solitary suffering, and within which his – and my – symmetric undifferentiated sensations could be clad in thought.

And thus I had occasion to say to Mike, with sincerity, "Thank you so much."

An unexpected clearing where everything happens at once

Blending the two epigrams that open this chapter, I can say that in my work with Mike, we became lost together in the flow of the symmetric enactment and found ourselves in an unexpected clearing where, as is the case when one enters the infinite spaces where time and space are melted, everything happened at once.

Here I am utilizing the precious theorizing offered by Matte Blanco and Lombardi, who have opened our eyes to this dimension of intrapsychic functioning where we touch infinity. Rather than seeking to move Mike out of "a dangerous timelessness" (Lombardi, 2016, p. 165) and into time-oriented reality, I anticipate that this dimension of his intrapsychic functioning will pervade the field and will engage me in ways that I could not possibly predict. Hence I do not seek to impede the emergence of this symmetric enactment and introduce asymmetry, but rather remain unobtrusive to its full phenomenological expression within and between both of us. I have surrendered myself to the flow of a mutual enactment of symmetric logic where we both find ourselves together in timelessness and spacelessness.

When he arrived for his session some weeks before in a disoriented, diffuse state where symmetric logic pervaded his perceptions such that he asked me to remember his unremembered dream, I did not seek to curtail or control this state but remained unobtrusive to the emerging expression of the symmetric state in the field of the treatment. It is my contention that such an unobtrusive companioning of the patient within this emergent symmetric enactment does not plunge the patient further into a lost world of boundarilessness, indistinctness, and psychosis – quite the opposite. I suggest that when accompanied and recognized in this space, the bounty of bi-logic, the interweaving of asymmetric logic and the personal truth of symmetry, can emerge and take hold within the patient and in the field. Furthermore, this unfolding will be imprinted with the stamp of the patient's – and the specific analytic couple's – very own creativity and personality, rather than learned from the authority that the analyst is supposed to know (Lacan, 2016).

Thus, some weeks later, when I was shivering during his morning session, Mike found himself able to utilize the benefits of symmetric tendency with great empathy for my bodily and mental state, responding to the "sensation-sentiment" (Lombardi, 2016, p. 11) of the moment, along with the developing asymmetric qualities of distinctness and difference such that he recognized that I was cold while he was not. If Mike found himself in a timeless zone some weeks before when he asked if I could remember his dream – evoking the earliest merged relation of an infant and mother – then I found myself in a timeless zone where an arcane and painful part of my emotional life was evoked when he responded to my silent suffering as I shivered in my chair. Everything was happening at once. If I found Mike when I told him that I wished I could remember his dream, then he could find a long dormant part of me when he responded bi-logically to my shivering. Thus, we had both become lost in a mutual timeless and spaceless symmetric enactment and were both found in surprising clearings that emerged unbidden in the companioned flow of that enactment. Greater differentiation within his mind emerged from being companioned in symmetric fusion.

We were both immersed in "Jewish time," moving "frontward to the past" (Oz & Oz-Salzberger, 2012, p. 118).

Notes

1 I wish to thank the reading group I attend with Donnel Stern, PhD, for helping me formulate my ideas for this chapter: Lisa Director, Orna Guralnik, Arthur Heiserman, Katherine Leddick, James Ogilvie, Debbie Rothschild, Liz Weiss.
2 For those interested, I would recommend, in addition to Matte Blanco's own writings (1975, 1988), the renditions of Lombardi (2016), Rayner (1995), and Rayner and Tuckett (1988).
3 The concept of the "basic matrix" evokes Loewald's (1978) concept of "primordial density" as the signature of primary process.
4 This inner flow of bi-logic where symmetrical and asymmetrical logic interweave resonates with the Bionian image of the constant interplay and imbrication of paranoid-schizoid and depressive position functioning.
5 Clinically, we find pockets of symmetrical logic in ordinary, "neurotic" presentations. For instance, Lombardi (2016) points to the catastrophic, infinite terror and loss of sense of time and context in panic attacks. In fact, one might say that panic attacks involve a momentary immersion in symmetric logic, and that is exactly why they can be so terrifying.
6 Recall the intensive motility exhibited by Kyle (Chapter 1), Bernard (Chapter 3), and Lloyd (Chapter 4).
7 Both Matte Blanco and Lombardi recognize that symmetric logic contains the elements that contribute to the development of empathy when integrated in bi-logic.
8 I should note that my colleague Debbie Rothschild, PhD, told me that on that very same morning she was subject to exactly the same thermostatic dilemma in her office and that she had spent the morning wrapped in the blanket she keeps in her office. Unlike me, she was thus not cold. However, some of her patients, seeing her wrapped in a blanket, feared that she was sick. Ah well: One is never not in an enactment, is one?

References

Alvarez, A. (1992). *Live company: Psychoanalytic psychotherapy with autistic, borderline, deprived and abused children.* London: Routledge.

Amis, M. (1991). *Time's arrow: Or the nature of the offense.* London: Jonathan Cape.

Balint, M. (1968). *The basic fault.* London; New York: Bruner/Mazel Publishers.

Bion, W. R. D. (1950). The imaginary twin. In *Second thoughts* (pp. 3–22). London: Karnac Books.

Bion, W. R. D. (1967). *Second thoughts: Selected papers on psycho-analysis.* Northvale, NJ: Jason Aronson.

Freud, S. (1900). The interpretation of dreams. In J. Strachey (Ed. & Trans.), *The standard edition of the complete psychological works of Sigmund Freud* (Vol. 4/5, pp. 1–627). London: Hogarth Press.

Freud, S. (1915). The unconscious. In J. Strachey (Ed. & Trans.), *The standard edition of the complete psychological works of Sigmund Freud* (Vol. 14, pp. 159–215). London: Hogarth Press.

Freud, S. (1940). An outline of psychoanalysis. In J. Strachey (Ed. & Trans.), *The standard edition of the complete psychological works of Sigmund Freud* (Vol. 23, pp. 139–208). London: Hogarth Press.

Green, A. (1986). *On private madness.* London: Hogarth Press.

Katz, G. (2014). *The play within the play: The enacted dimension of psychoanalytic process.* London: Routledge.

Lacan, J. (2016). *The seminar of Jacques Lacan, book X.* Cambridge: Polity Press.

Loewald, H. W. (1978). Primary process, secondary process, and language. In J. H. Smith (Ed.), *Psychoanalysis and language* (pp. 178–206). New Haven, CT: Yale University Press.

Lombardi, L. (2016). *Formless infinity: Clinical explorations of Matte Blanco and Bion.* London: Routledge.

Lombardi, R. (2002a). Primitive mental states and the body: A personal view of Armando Ferrari's concrete original object. *International Journal of Psychoanalysis, 83,* 363–381.

Lombardi, R. (2002b). Through the eye of the needle: Unfolding of the unconscious and the body. In *Formless infinity: Clinical explorations of Matte Blanco and Bion* (pp. 62–87). London: Routledge.

Matte Blanco, I. (1975). *The unconscious as infinite sets.* London: Karnac Books.

Matte Blanco, I. (1988). *Thinking, feeling and being: Clinical reflections on the fundamental antinomy of human beings and world.* London: Routledge.

Oz, A., & Oz-Salzberger, F. (2012). *Jews and words.* New Haven, CT: Yale University Press.

Rayner, E. (1995). *Unconscious logic: An introduction to Matte Blanco's bi-logic and its uses.* London: Routledge.

Rayner, E., & Tuckett, D. (1988). An introduction to Matte Blanco's reformulation of the Freudian unconscious and his conceptualization of the internal world. In

I. Matte Blanco, *Thinking, feeling and being: Clinical reflections on the fundamental antinomy of human beings and world* (pp. 3–42). London: Routledge.

Reis, B. (2009). We: Commentary on papers by Trevarthen, Ammaniti & Trentini, and Gallese. *Psychoanalytic Dialogues, 19*, 565–579.

Stern, D. B. (1997). *Unformulated experience: From dissociation to imagination in psychoanalysis.* Hillsdale, NJ: The Analytic Press.

Transtromer, T. (1987). The clearing. In R. Haas (Ed.), *Tomas Transtromer: Selected poems* (p. 139). Hopewell, NJ: Ecco Press.

White, R. W. (1959). Motivation reconsidered: The concept of competence. *Psychological Review, 66*, 297–333.

Chapter 7

The work of the narrative and enactive co-narration

Simply put, narrative is *the representation of an event or a series of events*.

——(H. Porter Abbott, 2008, p. 13)

We know in our bones that stories are *made*, not *found* in the world.

—Jerome Bruner (2002, p. 23)

Narrative animals

What makes us human? Over the centuries, there have been multiple answers and conjectures in response to this question. One recurring answer, from the Bible to Plato and Aristotle and onward, is that what makes us human is our innate ability to tell and live stories. We are narrative animals (Gottschall, 2013; Gottschall & Wilson, 2005), making narratives as we imagine, experience, and dream. We confront the moments of our lives – whether banal, such as making a cup of coffee, or extraordinary, such as flying to the moon – as part of narrative, our own personal narrative and that of the species, our "narrative identity" (Ricouer, 2012, p. 199). Narrative is the "central function or instance of the human mind" (Jamison, 1981, p. 13). Other species do not seem to have this ability, although our forebears, the more developed primates, evidence the basic elements of narrative: sequence, connection, and links. We live in a world of narrative that is personally constructed. Our own memories are more guided by the rules of narrative than by "the facts." Narrative creates coherence and meaning out of the chaos, unpredictability, and unruliness of our experience and our lives. As Donnel Stern (2010) says: "Without narrative, affect would be chaotic and rudderless, as shapeless as a collapsed tent: and without affect, narrative would be dry and meaningless" (p. 117).

The ability to narrate is central to the formation and maintenance of human bonds and human community. The ability to understand that humans are driven by their own motivations, that people have minds and consciousness and that one thing follows from another, are not only the threads that bind the individual human mind within itself, but also link the individual to a shared reality and to community and cooperation. Likewise, that very connectedness and community is the wellspring of narrative itself. We are born into narrative.

Narrative is not simply a genetic given, although our propensity for it is found across all humans and all time. It is born and reborn every generation when mothers and infants interact. When a mother responds to her baby's shift in state and metabolizes that sensation, deducing without a moment's hesitation whether baby is cold, hungry, uncomfortable, or simply seeking contact, she is engaging with the human narrative story, and baby is learning the rudiments of what will make the world and others knowable and reachable (Demir et al., 2015). These early "proto-conversations" (Brazelton, 1993) carry inordinate amounts of information and are the building blocks of what will become character, identity, emotional connection, and motivation. Every single instance in this human drama is unique and, while adhering to genetic mapping, has its own register, character, and hue. We humans are thus narrative creatures, and narrative itself emerges in human interaction, in the "dyadic states of consciousness" shared by mother and baby (Tronick, 2001, 2003). What develops is "cooperative intersubjectivity" (Trevarthen, 2001), and narrative is intimately woven in as mother and baby enjoy their "relational emotions" (Trevarthen, 2001) in "communicative musicality" (Malloch & Trevarthen, 2009).

When this organic process of emergence of self and narrative identity is disrupted by ongoing developmental trauma and neglect, coherence of self is wounded and impeded and the primary coordinates of time, space, and self are dislodged. Life becomes infused with the "familiar chaos" (D. B. Stern, 1997) of rigidity and repetition. There is no next, only a repetitive present.

Abbott (2008) regards narrative as any "representation of an event or a series of events" (p. 13), and in so doing, he links the human narrative instinct to the equally definitive propensity to represent. Hence when narrative is interrupted, representation falters and we find ourselves in the territory of the unformulated (D. B. Stern, 1997) and the unrepresented (Levine et al., 2013). Thus, patients who have suffered trauma and developmental disruptions in the narrative of the self are unable to represent that very trauma until there is an Other with whom the narrative can emerge and find an address. This is the work of the narrative and enactive co-narration that I address in this chapter.

The substance of enactment and transformational co-narration

Narrative is far more than that which is spoken and conveyed in words. Roland Barthes (1966) suggests that "the narratives of the world are numberless" and "able to be carried by articulated language, spoken or written, fixed or moving images, gestures and the ordered mixture of all these substances" (p. 251). In psychoanalysis, we have tended to rely on the substance of "articulated language," the tellable and the relatable. But the broader and multiple sense of narrative invites that which cannot be told and that which can only find expression via other "substances" such as gestures and behaviors and, if you will, the eloquence of action. I think here of Davidson and Malloch (2009) who speak of "gestural narratives" (p. 565) and Daniel Stern (2004) who evokes "lived non-verbal stories." To these narrative substances I add enactment. Enactment, as I understand it, always involves both analyst and patient together – and all members of a group – and the emergent field.[1] Hence in mutual enactment we find the emergence and arising of narratives that hitherto had no form or representation and therefore could not have been told in language. They come to be "told" in the register of mutual enactment, what I will term *enactive co-narration*. The unrepresented needs space to emerge and grow in the treatment, and the work of the unobtrusive relational analyst is to know that he or she will inevitably play an essential part in making what had hitherto been unthinkable come to life. We strive to let the fertile "germinative soil" (Neri, 1998, p. 23) of the analytic field do its work and to not obtrude. To intrude and examine it precipitously would be rather like pulling up a plant to look at the roots in order to see how it is growing.[2]

This participatory living-through together is itself a transformative element of psychoanalysis: a transformation from a no-thing to a potential and then to a something, a narrative. This is narrative that cannot be known or represented until it has been lived through with an Other. The fragmented, digital (Bach, 2008) pieces of potential self are drawn together into a narrative. A coherent story emerges as it is lived through with the analyst and in that living through becomes thinkable. The digital is transformed into the analogic (Bach, 2008) via "transformational co-narration" (Ferro, 2006, p. 1) of analyst and patient.

From his neo-Bionion perspective, Ferro (2006) describes how transformational co-narration creates meaning out of disparate pieces of beta elements. We must "be able to let ourselves be contaminated with the 'material' of (the patients') narrations and to go where it takes us" (p. 4). We must enter the patients' worlds on their terms, using their "narremes" (p. 4), their idiom. Ferro is largely talking about verbally conveyed pieces of potential meaning, the "narremes" of the patient and the field. I extend the concept of transformational co-narration to include the registers of the motoric and somatic as well as the enigmatic substance of mutual enactment in enactive co-narration.

The teller and the told

For a story to exist, "there needs to be a narrator, a teller, and there needs to be a listener or reader, a told" (Bruner, 2002, p. 17). Once there is a told, a participating receiver – imagined or real, someone to make the story with the teller – then there is a next. When there is a next, time and narrative come to life, the frozenness of trauma begins to thaw and the most fundamental question, basic to every narrative emerges: "What happens next?" This is the subjunctivizing of reality (Bruner, 2002) that heralds the kindling of reflection, agency, and perspective.

The image of the teller and the told affirms the ethos of mutual co-narration and Bruner's credo, included as the epigraph to this chapter, that stories are made, not found. We humans are narrative creatures, and as such we seek others with whom we can make our narratives. More than simply an other to *receive* the already formulated narrative, we seek the Other with whom we can *make* the narrative, to be the co-narrator. Meaning, Donnel Stern (1997) tells us, is made, not given. And so it is with narrative.

Donnel Stern (2010) emphasizes that it is the creation of new possible narratives that emerge in the relatedness between patient and analyst that foment change rather than from the analyst's objective interpretation of the patient's narrative as Schafer (1983, 1992) and Spence (1982, 1987) had suggested. Stern places the creation of new narrative freedom at the center of the therapeutic action of psychoanalysis and foregrounds the human need for a witness with whom to create narrative out of chaos. Beautifully rendering the isolation of those who seek witness to their trauma – the stories of Robinson Crusoe and the Incredible Shrinking Man – he emphasizes the human need to find or create a witness, either real or imagined, who will see, listen, and recognize the experience so that "once the isolated trauma sufferer gains a witness, the experience of the trauma becomes more possible to know, feel and think about"(D. B. Stern, 2010, p. 110). Without a witness – or as Stern puts it, a partner in thought – there is no story at all "*until something happens in ongoing relatedness* that allows us to see that someone else recognizes the pain we ourselves have been unable to know and feel" (p. 114, my emphasis). In this way, the Told creates the Teller such that empty non-experience becomes a narrative. It is the something that "happens in ongoing relatedness" that creates narrative where there had been none before that is the subject of this chapter.

Stern describes the "narrative freedom" that emerges in a "continuous productive unfolding" (pp. 116–118) as the treatment progresses. From Stern's perspective, this productive process is interrupted by enactment. Enactment occurs when a dissociated state in the patient "calls out a dissociated or not-me state in the analyst" (p. 121). This is a mutual enactment that rigidifies clinical relatedness and "interrupts each person's capacity to serve as witness for the other"; "events remain coded in procedural terms, in action" (p. 123).

From the perspective of enactive co-narration, these enactments are not seen as interruptions in the unfolding narrative but are the emergence of narrative in the register of non-representation. In other words, what is being represented is the failure of representation itself along with the content of that failed representation. The narrative does continue to emerge but in the register of action – eloquent or otherwise – in the procedural and somatic, or, blending Barthes, via the substance of enactment.

I lean here on Reis's (2009) concept of "enactive witnessing" that regards psychoanalytic witnessing as the "living out of traumatic experiences in the consulting room" rather than "having to do with warded-off dissociated self-states" (p. 1360). Hence the trauma is a "relational event" (p. 1363) that "comes to reside in the transference-countertransference matrix through various forms of action performed and enacted in the dyad" (p. 1359). Furthermore, adopting an analytic attitude very close to that of the unobtrusive relational analyst, Reis suggests that the analyst must "allow and witness memory in its varied forms, without attempting to symbolize or make personally understandable the experience – to accept the experience of the experience of trauma, without therapeutic ambition" (p. 1360). Like the unobtrusive relational analyst, Reis is urging us to allow the space for a mutual enactment of trauma that must unfold and become realized in its own time and register. Thus, it is the work of the analyst to be unobtrusive and to companion the patient in the emergence of the non-symbolized and non-mentalized enactive co-narration of trauma and of character. Both analyst and patient become teller and told together.

Psychoanalysis, action, and memory

Freud (1914) famously considered that repeating in action is a form of remembering and many have addressed the issue of action in regard to memory. The emphasis of psychoanalytic cure has predominantly been on the role of interpretation to transform the primary process world of thing (and therefore action) representations into secondary process and word representation. However, in recent years, there has been a growing appreciation of the role of enactment in psychoanalysis (Katz, 2014). It was Hans Loewald (1980) who differentiated "enactive remembering" and "representational remembering" (p. 164). He included acting out, transference, and "identificatory reproductions" in the former and verbal recollections in the latter (p. 164). Further, he equated enactive remembering with unconscious process and representational remembering with preconscious or conscious processes. For Loewald, this did not simply mean that "enactive remembering" implies that the patient has no awareness of the enactment of the memory (as when a patient does not simply describe his father's behavior but acts as if he *is* the father in the session), but such unconscious remembering "shares the timelessness and lack of differentiation of the unconscious and of the primary process"[3] (p. 165) such that "instead of *having* a past, (the patient) *is* his past and does not distinguish himself as a rememberer from the content of his memory" (p. 165).

Loewald was writing before the contemporary embrace of field theory in psychoanalysis and the awakening of relational theory and the foregrounding of intersubjectivity and mutual enactment. But if we integrate his prescient ideas in the current discussion, from the enactive co-narration approach of this chapter, when we allow ourselves to unobtrusively enter the patient's world and allow the field to flourish, the patient and analyst together *become* the patient's past – the past is lived in the treatment via "identificatory reproductions" on the part of both patient and analyst in a form of mutual "enactive remembering." In so doing, together with the patient we create "links of action" (Loewald, 1980, p. 169), which create meaning – *in themselves* – in the register of action. The remarkable suggestion here is that narration of trauma and of the patient's identifications and internal world take place entirely unconsciously to both parties in the register of action. This is a register that resides outside of language and cognition and perhaps needs to remain unknowable. This is a register that Christopher Bollas (2011) addresses with his concept of "interformality."

The remarkable rendezvous

Recall Abbott's suggestion in the epigram of this chapter that narration is a representation of an event. In psychoanalysis, then, enactive co-narration is a co-representation. And what is represented in the co-narrated emergent field is trauma, and beyond trauma, it is self. Together, the analyst and patient co-create the narrative of what has yet to have shape, and for so many of our patients that is nothing less than the narration of their selves.

Christopher Bollas (2009) argued for a drive to represent the self, for the "pleasure principle of self discovery and of being understood" (p. 37) in an analysis where the patient's being is articulated as a form of expression. Character is form and is irreducible. The work of analysis involves the reciprocal meeting of the characters of analyst and patient in what Bollas (2011) terms "interformality." This is the zone "where thoughts arrive as actions," where language has its limitations, where presentation is foregrounded over representation and where knowledge is derived from doing rather than talking: "To act is to realize" (p. 239). Language can convey content, but form and essence are not reducible to language. Interformality involves the real of the patient meeting the real of the analyst. Such deep connection cannot be translated into the symbolic or the imaginary.

It seems to me that Bollas is describing a register of psychoanalytic engagement that invites the unfolding of the narrative of the self in actions and the area of relatedness that cannot be translated into verbal understanding. He calls this "character association" that imparts the "idiom of the analysand's being and relating through the sequence and idiom of actions" (p. 243). Furthermore, his concept of interformality would seem to capture the unsymbolizable connection between patient and analyst that emanates from the depth of each of their characters as in Loewald's "enactive remembering." Each analytic pair will therefore have a unique idiom of narration, "a remarkable rendezvous of two irreducible natures is accomplished" (p. 247).

From the perspective of this chapter, I take Bollas to be underscoring the value of letting the narrative of actions, of the real, speak as they emerge in the enactive co-narration of the analytic couple. This is the narration of the self as form in engagement with the form of the analyst. I borrow from Bollas and suggest that when the unobtrusive relational analyst can companion the patient in unfolding emergent enactive co-narration, "without therapeutic ambition" (Reis, 2009, p. 1360), we witness a "remarkable rendezvous" where what had no form or content comes to be realized in mutual action and where the patient's self comes to be expressed as form. Enactment is narration in the real.

Two examples

The rest of this chapter is devoted to the detailed description of two cases that illustrate the work of the narrative and enactive co-narration. The work of the analyst is to be unobtrusive to the work of the narrative, such that the mutual enactive co-narration can unfold and take its own shape and form, can tell its own story in the real. The first case, Pamela, highlights the enacted co-narration of a traumatized and traumatizing relationship. This enacted co-narration makes real and emotionally present an aspect of Pamela's life that she knew as an ongoing reality but could gain no emotional purchase on. This left her locked in a repetitive life without agency, trapped in a false self. The narrative emerges in the field with the unconscious participation of both patient and analyst. Both are teller and told simultaneously. The second case, Nick, tells of the unfolding enactive co-narration of early trauma. This trauma was not known or even thought of by Nick but it had a powerful and defining influence on his symptomatology and character. The field comes to be the teller and the told of what had yet to have form. In both these cases, the enactive co-narration unfolds. Change comes from the living through of these moments companioned by the analyst. In the case of Pamela, the enactment is recognized and processed in the clinical process. In the case of Nick, its location in the realm of enactment, the realm "where thoughts arrive as actions" (Bollas, 2011,

p. 238), of "links of action" (Loewald, 1980), is respected and related to as such. In both cases, the enactment involves something "that happens in ongoing relatedness" (D. B. Stern, 2010) that transforms the patient, the treatment, and the analytic couple forever.

Pamela[4]

Pamela, a small, attractive 25-year-old Latin-American woman, had been referred by the counseling center at her college where she was completing a graduate degree in business systems technology. She spoke of sadness after an unsuccessful relationship, a long struggle with depression, difficulty sleeping, and a lifelong feeling that "the cards are stacked against me"; "I'm defeated before I even begin." She spoke with a clarity and urgency of the insecure part of her and the angry part of her that "don't talk to each other." "This causes me pain," she said, "I can't even talk about it. I just don't have the words." She complained that the therapist she saw previously for about two years was very silent. She had left that therapy in a rage when he forgot some facts about her job that she had described at length to him in a previous session. I gathered that being forgotten and ignored would be a central part of her treatment. She commented that she felt "comforted" that I was taking notes as she spoke. Having this concrete evidence that, at least so far, I was paying attention, she proceeded to give some images of her family.

Both Pamela's parents had emigrated from the country of their birth in Central America via various countries and in different ways had been ravaged by years of war and destruction in their homeland. Her father's father had been murdered when her father was a teenager. Her father would never talk about why this happened, but rumors of betrayal and shame hung in the family air. Her mother had lost two brothers and various uncles and cousins. Some have reappeared; others are presumed dead or gone forever. After much struggle and suffering, the couple had found their way to the US with her mother's mother and some cousins and had made a home in a Midwestern city. The father had worked hard at various business ventures and had, after some failures, set up an industrial cleaning supply distribution business that had become very successful. Pamela's mother did not work but helped out in the business when she was needed. Pamela and her brother had been brought up in the tight quarters of a small home and within their first years saw the family prosper and move into a large house and affluent neighborhood.

Pamela was quite clear that she could never tell her parents that she was in therapy. They would never understand. She described a deep parental preference for her brother, the male child. He went to private school, she to public. He was urged to follow a career; they grumbled and just about accepted her desire to go to college. Pamela described how she has forever felt a constant anger and shame. Everything has been a battle.

It became clear during the sessions that followed that she had developed sophisticated social and personal skills to make her way in the world. She was a smart and efficient worker in her field, and when she finished graduate school soon after she began treatment, she was able to secure a well situated and quite demanding management position. She had a full and busy social life and was often the "go-to" friend, the one to organize the parties, summer houses, and trips. She was popular, dynamic, and attractive. She seemed to have little difficulty in drawing attention from men she would desire and on the outside seemed to be living the New York single life to the fullest.

In her sessions, she gradually revealed that she lived in a hell, a war zone. She felt slighted by the smallest things and would plunge into attacks on herself and on those who she saw as culpable. In her mind, she would castigate the guilty with a cutting arrogance and haughtiness. Alternatively, even the most innocuous slight could cut her to the core. She could be devastated by anyone and anything. She felt unbearable shame. She would attack and criticize herself mercilessly for being so vulnerable and weak.

Pamela's emotions and her body were dysregulated. She complained that emotions overwhelmed her. She was powerless in the face of the onslaught of her own anger, sadness, and confusion: "The emotion – it comes on me in a wave. Uncontrollable. Overwhelming." She was frequently unable to make sense of things and sort out her emotional reality: "How do I take in what I need and leave what I don't need? I have no filter. No boundary. No ability to discriminate." Her body was beset by pain. She had chronic back pain, digestive problems diagnosed as Irritable Bowel Syndrome, and headaches.

She seemed to have nothing to hold on to in life except for the sensation of her own emotions flowing through her. She would feel grounded and protected by anger and hate. Sorrow also seemed to regulate her; she would play sad music so that she would be able to cry herself to sleep at night. She was in tremendous emotional pain and said, "This body, it's just too small to carry all this pain." And indeed it seemed to me that she carried the pain and trauma of her own life and that of previous generations.

At first, she was scared of what treatment would open up for her and wanted to come only once per week. She feared that neither she nor I could handle what she felt she carried inside. It took some months before she trusted the treatment enough to come two times per week and many more months before she settled into three sessions per week. She paid for the treatment herself, using her earned income.

During those first months, a picture emerged of a family with no boundaries and no ability to contain virtually any emotion. The parents would scream and rage at each other, never seeming to share a kind or loving word. They would complain to the children about each other. Bathroom doors would never be closed no matter whether they were washing or defecating. The parents were often in various states of undress around the house.

Her mother would criticize the smallest things that Pamela did: how she walked, where she sat, and what she talked about. She would be yelled at frequently and only sometimes did she understand why. She was perpetually confused and fearful. When the anger spilled over, severe beatings were meted out to the children. It took some years for Pamela to put together a narrative of the punishments and beatings. The most painful aspect for her is that she rarely did anything wrong. She was a good, obedient girl. But her brother would do something to spark the parents' fury, and both would be summarily punished. She often had no clue what had happened. The children would suddenly be dragged into the bathroom that was in the center of the house. It was the room with no windows onto the outside. You couldn't see into it, and no one on the outside could hear you scream: a torture chamber. There would be spankings and hitting and then when she was trapped in the corner the whip would come out. She'd try to fight back, make herself impervious to the pain. During one period of treatment, Pamela would experience a pain in the outside of her forearm during sessions. It was some time before we put together the idea that she used to raise her arm to protect herself from the blows raining down on her and that her forearm would take the brunt of the blows. No one in the family seemed to be able to contain their rage or fears. Pamela remembers one occasion when in the heat of a disagreement with her father he grabbed the sharpest kitchen knife, pointed it at his stomach, and screamed at Pamela to kill him right there and then. On another occasion, her mother, too, taunted her with not being able to kill her, the mother. Her grandmother who lived with them seems to have been a massively traumatized person herself. She had lost two sons in their country. When overwhelmed with anger or grief or just sheer frustration – Pamela doesn't know which – she would bang her head against the wall while in the company of Pamela and her brother.

Coupled with the terror, confusion, and pain of the household was the neglect that Pamela suffered. She has many memories of being forgotten about. Often she would be left after school and not picked up. Her birthday passed without anyone remembering on more than one occasion. One particularly painful memory is of her desperate efforts to assure that her mother would be available to drive her to her best friend's eagerly anticipated birthday party, only for the time to arrive and for there to be no one at home. Time passed and finally, much too late, her mother arrived only to utter a glib, "Oh, but I had to do some shopping."

Pamela tried everything to get some kind of attention as a child. She remembers leaving notes around the house saying that she hated her mother and was going to kill her and that she was going to kill herself. She constantly thought of suicide. No one said anything. She told me a dream in which she was a child asleep, clutching her blanket, on a traffic island in the middle of a busy street with cars zooming past on all sides. She is totally alone and unprotected.

She did, however, get attention from her father. Alongside his participation in the abuse and neglect, he treated her as his "special little girl" and adored her. He would shower her with special gifts, and she recalls her mother's dark disappointment and envy when this would happen. He told Pamela that she reminded him of his mother whom he adored. She says that she always sensed that he had some kind of sexual feelings toward her, yet is sure there was never any actual sexual contact. As a child, she was pleased to be the preferred one, to be "Daddy's Little Girl" and to displace her mother, who her father relentlessly criticized. This all ended abruptly when she reached middle school and became obviously depressed. "If I wasn't happy and adoring, he seemed to have no place for me."

There were terrors outside the home as well as inside. They were the only family of color in their town, and she has painful memories of being taunted and sadistic tricks being played on her by some fellow students.

Pamela found a way to survive. She took radical control of her body and her environment. She became obsessively clean and organized in her room and always shut her bedroom door. She found comfort in the Church and for most of her teenage years maintained an involvement there.

She became perfect as a student, excelling in her schoolwork and extra-curricular activities. She also became perfect as a friend and developed her ability to be pleasing and charming (a version of the sweet and charming little girl who had initially secured her father's attention). She was always available to help and organize. She made friends with the coolest and most attractive kids in school and described how she always lived with an intense anxiety that she would be unmasked in some way. She would then redouble her efforts at perfection.

With boys, and later with men, she produced the Perfect Pamela. Nothing was too much. She attracted the most sought after boys, and later wealthy and dynamic men. She would typically grow frustrated that she was giving everything and receiving little, and eventually feel misunderstood and abused. Sexually she felt little arousal herself. She felt that, inside, she didn't yet have adult sexual feelings. She felt either pain during sex or nothing much at all and was totally focused on delivering pleasure for the man. It was some years into treatment before she began to dream of being held and feeling comfortable with a man, and some further time before she began to enjoy and take pleasure in sex.

Some time into the treatment, she dreamed that she was in a dark cave looking for someone. "But I was looking for me. I saw this little person crying, wriggled up in a ball, crying. I reached out to help and the child bit me. My first reaction was to yell, but eventually I held the child while it screamed. The child gradually calmed down." This dream seemed to accurately capture her self and seemed to describe what she needed from treatment, to not be yelled at, but to be found and held, despite her biting rage.

Indeed, I tried to provide a stable and containing environment where she could sort through the swirl of emotions that enveloped her and to find her self and her pain. I would also have to survive some intense "biting." She was helped to feel grounded in the treatment by taking charge of the room in her own way. She would always require a cushion at her lower back for support, and the clock was to be placed where she could see it. At various times she has been on the couch, in different chairs and positions, but these elements have always been in place.

As we progressed, she constructed a meaningful narrative and made connections that seemed to bring relief. However, I was beset with a feeling that I can best describe as the sense that this was not really real. I would be surprised to find myself bored and distracted. In time, she began to articulate that she often slipped into states where she did not exist. She said, "I'll be in a conversation with people and I'll worry maybe I'm not real, I'm not here . . . to feel you're in a room, but you're not . . . no one sees you or hears you, I'm so frightened, I'll get light-headed . . . none of this is real, it's a movie or something . . . I'll be in the shower and suddenly the water feels a bit different, then it's like I'm watching a movie. I'm not in my own body. I'll touch my arm, and I can't feel I'm being touched. I'm losing my memory. I'll forget to put my contact lenses in. I'll begin to panic and I'll say to myself 'calm down, it's OK' and I'll try to focus on what I need to do today, to organize my thoughts."

In time, she would have these experiences in and around her sessions. For some years we have grappled with what it is like to have been killed repeatedly. She is clear that while the actual physical trauma of the beating was bad, more than anything it is that she was emotionally killed. She has had to face the terror, or the "abyss" as she calls it, of being dead, of having not existed.

Of course, the horror emerged in enactive co-narration in the treatment. On occasion, she has caught me not listening with the attention she required. Her rage is intense and "biting." She knows how to beat someone. And then there was the time I "killed" her: an enactive co-narration of psychic murder. Pamela was away for some weeks on vacation, and I received a call from a woman who described herself as an acquaintance of Pamela's. She said that Pamela had recommended me to her as an analyst. We arranged a consultation after I felt I had ascertained on the phone that she was not a close friend of Pamela's. We met for an initial consultation. On Pamela's return, she was in a violent rage. "How could you have met with Teresa?" she screamed. I was horrified and realized, as I heard the name come out of her mouth, that this was indeed a friend of whom she had spoken much. Their relationship was complicated and competitive. "You're just like all the rest," she screamed, "I'm nothing to you. As soon as you can bring in more money, I'm shit. Nothing!" She decided there and then to end the treatment. I barely managed to pull myself together, reeling from the shock and the realization that I had conducted the whole consultation with Teresa in a dissociated state and had dropped Pamela from my mind, and thus psychically murdered her. I told her that I would not continue the consultation with Teresa and that I was mortified that I had done this. I told her, as the thoughts came to me: "My God: I became your mother and your father all at once." We managed over the following sessions to look at what had happened and how I had embodied her parents. I had functioned in a numbed state in which I went through the motions of an analyst without applying my mind and thinking carefully about what I was doing and the impact this might have on Pamela. I had lost her from my mind and effectively killed her and almost killed the treatment.

I think my sincerity and visible distress were crucial in helping her find the other parts of her that were able to maintain her connection to me and to stay in treatment and turn this enactment of potential murder into an experience of repair and recognition. More dreams followed of dead children being found and somehow revived, and the treatment was indeed revived. However, it was not until some months later, when she had a vivid dream of highly desirable designer Prada bags that were filled with shit, that she began to consider her participation in the episode with Teresa. She turned to me and with fear and wonder asked why she, Pamela, had given my name and number to Teresa. Until that moment, I had not quite held that question in my mind either: I had been so mortified by my own behavior. She sunk into the couch and in a quiet and matter-of-fact tone said that she knew that she herself was full of shit. She marveled at how she had created the conditions for her own murder in and of the treatment. Really, we concluded, it had been a moment of murder-suicide. It was as if she had held the sharp kitchen knife to her own belly and yelled at me to plunge it in – as her father had done with her – and I had complied. We had co-narrated various aspects of her emotional life: being murdered by being forgotten about by her mother; her identification with her enraged and destructive father; her identification with the evacuative quality of her mother's psychic make-up and with the sadomasochistic dimension of the parents' relationship; and her own rage at being diminished by both parents in their preference for her older brother and more. But what felt equally compelling was the weight she felt in her small body of carrying the family history of murders and what she now considered as probable suicides that had never been talked about. She spoke with quiet clarity and feeling that she was beginning to understand her grandmother's silent pain and anguish that could only be expressed through the self-harm of banging her head against the wall. The ghosts and demons of multi-generational trauma were announcing their presence in our enactive co-narration (Harris et al., 2016a, 2016b).

I look back now at this sequence of clinical events and marvel at the depth of narrative that emerged between us in this enactment that had, at first, caused me deep anguish. Indeed, my own pain and self-recriminations on realizing what I had wrought by consulting with Teresa were also a feature of this enactive co-narration. I too was carrying some of the unbearable pain that Pamela struggled to manage within her. Recall Ferro's (2006) suggestion that we must be able to let ourselves be "contaminated with the 'material' of (the patients') narrations" and "go where it takes us" (p. 4). That certainly feels accurate here. What also strikes me is the narrative quality of the enactment. Rather than see this enactment as the foreclosing of narrative, I see it as the very emergence of the necessary and previously unthought narrative that finally could speak via this enactive co-narration. Pamela and I seem to have conveyed the idiom of her very "being and relating through the sequence and idiom of actions" (Bollas, 2011, p. 243). We had narrated her character.

In Loewald's idiom, Pamela did not *have* her past; she *was* her past. Or, more accurately from the enactive co-narration approach of this chapter, Pamela and I *were* her past in a timelessness zone together where I came to *be* her parents and we came to live an "identificatory reproduction" of how she had been treated in her family. The links that created meaning were "links of action" (Loewald, 1980, p. 169). I would suggest that this could not have happened without our joint participation in the enactive co-narration.

For Pamela, this sequence in our relationship was transformative. After a sequence of relationships with men, she finally settled with a man who was kind to her. She was initially confused, never having experienced a boyfriend taking care of her rather than simply waiting for her to always be cute and caretaking herself. The relationship deepened, he proposed marriage and she accepted.

Having lived through the enacted co-narration of murder-suicide, the treatment relationship deepened immeasurably as did her own ability to care for herself. In addition to the greater sense of connection and safety with me in the treatment and the calm she felt with her fiancé, Pamela found other sources of holding and self-regulation. She began yoga classes and workshops and pursued weekly massage sessions with a bodywork practitioner. She became more located in her own body and in her own self.

She gradually revisited the experiences she had so long annulled by her all-too-efficient adaptation in life: She had been "not waving but drowning" (Smith, 1957) and no one, not even she, until now, had noticed. She confronted her mother about the abuse and persevered in the face of her mother's initial denial. She engaged her brother in long talks about their early experiences together, never before addressed, and found her father to be open to some frank moments concerning their mistakes as parents.

Nick[5]

Nick is a physicist in his early thirties who works in the pharmaceutical industry. Arriving in my office some years ago, he was an enraged ball of fury. His rage was directed at almost all authority and symbols of power. His superiors at work, the United States government, and anyone who did not see the world as he did were contemptuously derided. Those who stood up and fought the great evil were idealized and lauded, none more so than the 9/11 bombers and other suicidal fighters. I figured I had better just stay steady and try to create a safe space within which I could find out who this man was. I was aware that we were already in the realm of the enactive co-narration of disgust, repulsion, and violence. His hair and clothes were always unkempt and disorderly. They seemed to speak of a neglect and abandonment. Over time, he calmed down and articulated his difficulties with managing his emotions, his profound self-doubts, and the overwhelming rage that could leave him totally beside himself. The most comforting thing for him and for me in those first months of treatment was his dedication and devotion to his long-term girlfriend, who he described as a reliable and stable partner for him. Indeed, he also became dedicated to his treatment despite many periods of intense ambivalence and struggle.

He described his upbringing with a mix of pride and puzzlement. His parents raised Nick and his two brothers in a disorganized apartment in one of the city's housing projects. Nick's father was an inventor and a dreamer. The apartment was full of the father's inventions and jerry-rigged appliances and gizmos, many of which did not work and some of which were downright dangerous. He attempted to sell his inventions with little luck, and the family barely got by on the mother's occasional income as a sales assistant.

To myself, I questioned the sanity of his parents. Nick viewed his father as a pioneering dreamer type, a man among men, who would never compromise. His rage was mainly kept for his mother. She had left the home when he was five and had moved in with a sequence of other men and friends. He and his brothers subsequently lived an almost itinerant life, spending some time at the family apartment with their father and otherwise living in various households with the mother's lovers, her lovers' room-mates, and sometimes with people he simply could not place. He described how on one occasion around eight years old he was found scavenging for food in the garbage of a building he was staying in with another "aunt" whom he barely knew. He was dumb-struck when I suggested that he was neglected. It had never occurred to him.

His body and his sexuality were as chaotic as his rage. He believed for some of his teenage years that he was gay, tried to have sex with a close male friend, was promiscuous and hyper-stimulated with young girl-friends, and became fascinated with anuses and feces. We discussed the issue of sexual abuse and thought about possible suspects, mostly focusing on some of the men in the households in which he found himself staying when he was a child. He cannot recall anything specifically, but explicit sexual dreams involve his brothers, his friends, some of his caretakers, and so on. Like his body and his presentation, his mind and his memory were an evacuative mess of out of control images and stimulation. He was grounded and also traumatized by an obsession with child pornography. He was excited more than anything by the image of an innocent little girl who looks to be getting pleasure as she is sexually or violently abused. His descriptions of some of the websites that he would visit have at times been difficult for me to think about. Those explicitly involving screams, terror, and torture have caused me pain. I assume I am experiencing some part of his experience. The thing is, they all cause him immense pain, too.

He vigorously and seriously applied himself to his treatment, and I should say that I developed an affection and admiration for Nick. The courage it took for him to confront and talk about these living repetitive traumas was very compelling. He came to see that his child pornography obsession was a form of re-traumatization and self-assault, and he subsequently greatly decreased his use of the pornography. Yet the compulsion would continue to hold a real sway over him and he dreamed frequently of sexual activities with prepubescent girls as young as four or five. The dreams were extremely stimulating to him. He was living in a kind of hell. Sometimes being with him was a kind of hell for me, too. There were periods when the experience of our therapeutic inquiry collapsed into a concrete world where the integrity of his body and mind were severely challenged. There were explosive rages with me, and regressions where his talk disintegrated into word-salad ramblings and paranoid ideation. Once out of these states, he was often able to reorganize his mind and on occasion thanked me for my calm and caring during these episodes.

Over time, he responded to the holding and containment I tried to steadily provide, and he gradually opened up questions about who he really was. He began to question many beliefs he had taken on obsessively and passionately in his lifetime, including his anti-authoritarianism and his flirtation with homosexuality, among others. He worked hard to have relationships with both his parents and to accept and understand who they are and were while not avoiding anger and hurt that he still struggled with. He advanced in his career and, most powerfully, he married his girlfriend, and they had a baby boy, Billy, who was eight months old at the time of the session to be described below.

One day, he did not arrive on time for his session. He called after a time to say that the babysitter had not shown up due to sickness and that he had Billy with him and was stuck in traffic. He wasn't going to make it on time and inquired about a possible alternate time. I told him that I had a free hour some time later that day. He was happy about this and gratefully agreed to come then. He entered the office carrying Billy in the snuggly, and I helped him into the office with his book bag, his baby bag, his coat, and so on. First things first: Billy needed a change. Whether he requested my help or whether I simply began to assist, I do not know, but we worked together like a cohesive couple. Laying out the changing mat, changing the dirty diaper, I took on the role of assistant, removing the soiled diaper and wipes and helping him to locate this and that. I produced some toys and Sesame Street characters that I keep in my office closet. The room was filled with the sweet and shitty smell of baby poop. My office was transformed: furniture moved, smells, sights, and sounds swirling around. All the while, Nick cooed and played with Billy, and I couldn't resist a coo or two myself, becoming wrapped into the world of babyhood, that I had experienced fully only a couple of years prior with my own young children. I hadn't realized how much I missed it until then. Nick settled Billy into his lap and fed Billy as we settled into the session.

Nick told me a dream. And it was a horror. The switch from the nurturing environment we had constructed to the tortured abusive world of Nick's dream world was jarring and traumatic for me: the enacted co-narration of shock and abuse, and in the nursery, no less. In Nick's dream, vividly rendered in every detail, he found himself in potential sexual encounters with hyper-stimulating and seductive women whom he viewed as inappropriate and undesirable partners for him. The environment was soiled with excrement and vermin. He was, however, encouraged by the dream because in this dream he repeatedly recoiled from the women and refused to go along with the sex, aware of how sickening it felt.

While associating to the dream, there were intervals of tending to Billy. Both Nick and I played with the Sesame Street characters with Billy, and at one point kidded around with Elmo and Big Bird ourselves and enjoyed a chuckle together. At the end of the session, he settled Billy back into his snuggly, and I gathered the toys and put my office back together.

There is an enormous amount we could discuss about Nick: the chaos of his inner world; his constant dance with re-traumatization; the relationship between shit, shame, and defilement; the evacuative quality of thinking itself; and his search for containment and boundaries, which, to some degree, he found in the snuggly and the transitional play-space of the treatment.

However, the issue I wanted to draw our attention to here is the emergent enactive co-narration. The session began with a shifting of boundaries: On receiving Nick's call, I rescheduled the session there and then. As I realized that he was with Billy and running late, I consciously switched immediately into a mode of fellow father. I was in touch with that parent zone where surrender to the exigencies of care for young children simply overrides all else. I was able to be flexible and responsive even at some slight inconvenience to my own schedule and plan for the day. I think this is a kind of making do that parents engage in all the time. It is not the strict and rigid father of determination-at-all-costs that saw Nick's father plug away at his inventions to the point of ruination of his family's well-being, yet not a passive I'll-do-whatever-you-want father who neglects and avoids the issue of boundaries. Most importantly, I was responsive to a request that came in the form of action. Many analysts are wary of shifting and accommodating to patients' requests of this nature, often cleaving to the view that the boundary of the session time and place are sacrosanct. Although not aware of it at the time, I now consider that such requests are often the call to enter the world of the real, the "realm where thoughts arrive as actions" (Bollas, 2011, p. 239), and that our work involves unobtrusively responding to the call of that realm. It is the call of the narrative that can only find expression via self-presentation (Bollas, 2011) and action rather than spoken and dialogic representation. The denial of such a request, simply due to the psychoanalytic law of the father that says that the session can never be shifted when the frame does not fit the picture (Bass, 2007), might choke off the opportunity for the emergent enactive co-narration to unfold. Of course, I understand that one cannot simply comply with all patient requests, and that sometimes it would be deleterious to the treatment to do so. And, naturally, there are times when one simply cannot comply with patient requests because of ordinary logistical considerations. However, I am drawing our attention to the times when such a request is the manifestation of the patient's deep need to represent-with-an-other, to co-narrate what has yet to have any narrative or cognitive form in the patient's mind.

Consider the narratives that unfolded. Nick and I worked together to clean and accommodate a baby. We were male-moms together. We were partners. For me to share this kind of intimacy with Nick was very touching and enjoyable. I like babies and their care, and I think he was learning to. I also like this kind of intimacy with men, and it introduced a new register of intimacy into our relationship.[6] What seemed to emerge was a new space between us where we could play with this new and rare identity. And play we did, and with dolls, no less. A new "narrative identity" (Ricouer, 2012) was emerging in the register of doing.

And then came the enactive co-narration of sexual trauma, violence, and over-stimulation in the nursery when Nick shifted from our playful men-mom space into the horror of the dream. I should emphasize that in its telling Nick was not unduly upset or disrupted by the dream. He ploughed ahead with the telling of the dream and his associations to it. It was I who experienced the dark, violating horror of the dream. It was I who found it to be an almost impossible scene, to be holding a beautiful and content little six-month-old in one's arms while recounting such horror. My mind and spirit were the address where the trauma surfaced in the field. I experienced the horror of violation in that moment. As I struggled to maintain my own mental integrity in Nick's presence, I began to realize that we, our field, had narrated what could never be told because there was no teller: violation in the nursery. In fact, it is truer to say that there was a teller. But this teller was not an adult with access to verbal abilities and coherent dialogue. An infant cannot recount what has happened to him or her. But the mark of the violation endures. It was present in his painful, destructive symptoms of obsession with child pornography and his pedophilic dreams. But most tangibly, it emerged in the something "that happened in our ongoing relatedness" (D. B. Stern, 2010, p. 114). The teller was our joint enactive co-narration.

In the moment, I did not articulate these thoughts and observations. Nick was flowing in the session as he associated to the dream, and as I mentioned, he and I shifted states back and forth in the session, from the focus on the dream to the playful engagement with Billy. What was being narrated was not only the trauma, but the way in which the trauma had been encapsulated and managed. Hence I was left shuddering with the imprint of violation along with my earnest and truly enjoyable engagement with Billy and Nick and the Sesame Street characters. In terms of clinical process, I would not seek to intrude on this flow of narration with cognitive perspective when the session is flowing in this multi-layered way. To abruptly intrude would be to violate Nick's process and thereby shift the location of the violation to *his* being rather than allow it to sojourn in *mine*. It would have been a way to disgorge myself of the horror. I needed to hold it for safekeeping until the field and Nick could tolerate it. There would be plenty of time later to re-engage with the trauma. Indeed, we returned to the issue of childhood sexual abuse when some time later he dreamed that he was a small child and was being taken by the hand by a large adult and led down a path. The sense of the dream is foreboding. No memories have arisen to confirm or deny what actually happened, but it is safe to say that Nick believes that something of that nature must have happened, and he has accepted that he will probably never know for sure.

Rather than get snagged on the issue of whether or not such events actually took place, my purpose here is to illustrate how a welcoming unobtrusive relational analyst can flow with the patient and the field and allow for the enactive co-narration of personal truth. Nick was changed not by the revelation of probable abuse but, I would suggest, by the whole shift in ongoing relatedness that ensued between us. I include here the playfulness and parental-like cooperation as well as the emergent narrative of horror. In protecting the emergence of this joint narrative, I believe I protected the growth of a new narrative identity that felt more like his own personal truth.

Conclusion

I hope that the vignettes of my work with both Pamela and Nick have illustrated the thesis of this chapter that enactment may be usefully conceptualized as a form or register of narration and representation rather than a block in relatedness and the representational process of psychoanalysis. Further, it is a register that can be embraced and companioned by the analyst in the flow of enactive co-narration such that the work of the narrative can unfold and "speak" *in its own register*. Traumatic repetition becomes a communication (Reis, 2009) via "links of action" (Loewald, 1980).

The work of the narrative and enactive co-narration are ongoing and ever-present in all treatments. We are always enactively co-narrating with our patients. At times, it may go unremarked, but even a good therapeutic alliance may be regarded as the emergent co-narration of a successful attunement between mother and infant. Every patient and every session have their own character and shading, and the observant analyst will recognize the subtle or dramatic changes in one's self that inhere as one shifts from session to session as the day proceeds. These are the marks of shifts in enactive co-narrations with every one of our patients. Our work is to register these narratives and simultaneously to stay out of the way of their mutual unfolding. In politics, they say that to get to the truth one must follow the money. Perhaps in psychoanalysis we get closer to the truth if we follow the narrative.

Notes

1 See Chapters 9 and 10 for descriptions of unfolding narrative in group analysis.
2 I borrow this metaphor from the British poet Stevie Smith, who responded with this analogy when asked to describe her creative process (Poetry Please, 2017).
3 Notice the resonance between Loewald's formulation of enactive remembering and the timelessness and spacelessness of Matte Blanco's symmetric logic described in Chapter 6.
4 A longer version of this case was previously published as "The Case of Pamela" (Grossmark, 2009a).
5 A version of this case appears in Grossmark (2009b).
6 The issue of multiple masculinities and the many faces of intimacy between men are addressed in Reis and Grossmark (2009).

References

Abbott, H. P. (2008). *The Cambridge introduction to narrative (Cambridge introductions to literature)*. Cambridge, UK: Cambridge University Press.
Bach, S. (2008). On digital consciousness and psychic death. *Psychoanalytic Dialogues, 18*, 784–794.
Barthes, R. (1966). Introduction to the structural analysis of narratives. In S. Sontag (Ed.), *A Barthes reader* (p. 251). New York: Hill & Wang.

Bass, A. (2007). When the frame doesn't fit the picture. *Psychoanalytic Dialogues*, *17*, 1–27.

Bollas, C. (2009). Free association. In C. Bollas, *The evocative object world* (pp. 5–46). London: Routledge.

Bollas, C. (2011). Character and interformality. In C. Bollas, *The Christopher Bollas reader* (pp. 238–248). London: Routledge.

Brazelton, T. B. (1993). *Touchpoints: Your child's emotional and behavioral development*. New York: Viking.

Bruner, J. (2002). *Making stories: Law, literature and life*. Cambridge, MA: Harvard University Press.

Davidson, J., & Malloch, S. (2009). Musical communication: The body movements of performance. In S. Malloch & C. Trevarthen (Eds.), *Communicative musicality: Exploring the basis of human companionship* (pp. 565–583). Oxford: Oxford University Press.

Demir, O. E., Levine, S. C., & Goldin-Meadow, S. (2015). A tale of two hands: Children's early gesture use in narrative production predicts later narrative structure in speech. *Journal of Child Language*, *42*, 662–681.

Ferro, A. (2006). *Psychoanalysis as therapy and storytelling*. London, New York: Routledge.

Freud, S. (1914). Remembering, repeating and working-through. In J. Strachey (Ed. & Trans.), *The standard edition of the complete psychological works of Sigmund Freud* (Vol. 12, pp. 145–156). London: Hogarth Press.

Gottschall, J. (2013). *The story-telling animal: How stories make us human*. New York: Mariner Books.

Gottschall, J., & Wilson, D. S. (2005). *The literary animal: Evolution and the nature of narrative*. Chicago, IL: Northwestern University Press.

Grossmark, R. (2009a). The case of Pamela. *Psychoanalytic Dialogues*, *19*, 22–30.

Grossmark, R. (2009b). Two men talking. In B. Reis & R. Grossmark (Eds.), *Heterosexual masculinities: Contemporary perspectives from psychoanalytic gender theory* (pp. 73–87). New York: Routledge.

Harris, A., Kalb, M., & Klebanoff, S. (Eds.). (2016a). *Ghosts in the consulting room: Echoes of trauma in psychoanalysis*. London: Routledge.

Harris, A., Kalb, M., & Klebanoff, S. (Eds.). (2016b). *Demons in the consulting room: Echoes of genocide, slavery and extreme trauma in psychoanalytic practice*. London: Routledge.

Jamison, F. (1981). *The political unconscious: Narrative as a socially symbolic act*. Ithaca, NY: Cornell University Press.

Katz, G. (2014). *The play within the play: The enacted dimension of psychoanalytic process*. London: Routledge.

Levine, H. B., Reed, G. S., & Scarfone, D. (2013). *Unrepresented states and the construction of meaning: Clinical and theoretical contributions*. London: Karnac Books.

Loewald, H. (1980). Perspectives on memory. In H. Loewald, *Papers on psychoanalysis* (pp. 147–177). New Haven, CT: Yale University Press.

Malloch, S., & Trevarthen, C. (2009). *Communicative musicality: Exploring the basis of human companionship*. Oxford: Oxford University Press.

Neri, C. (1998). *Group*. London: Jessica Kingsley Publishers.

Poetry Please. (2017, May 27). *BBC World Service Radio Broadcast*.

Reis, B. (2009). Performative and enactive features of psychoanalytic witnessing: The transference as the scene of address. *International Journal of Psychoanalysis, 90*, 1359–1372.

Reis, B., & Grossmark, R. (Eds.). (2009). *Heterosexual masculinities: Contemporary perspectives from psychoanalytic gender theory*. New York: Routledge.

Ricouer, P. (2012). Life: A story in search of a narrator. In P. Ricouer, *On psychoanalysis* (pp. 187–200). Malden, MA: Polity Press.

Schafer, R. (1983). *The analytic attitude*. New York: Basic Books.

Schafer, R. (1992). *Retelling a life: Narration and dialogue in psychoanalysis*. New York: Basic Books.

Smith, S. (1957). *Not waving but drowning*. London: Andre Deutche Publishers.

Spence, D. (1982). *Narrative truth and historical truth: Meaning and interpretation in psychoanalysis*. New York: Norton.

Spence, D. (1987). *The Freudian metaphor: Toward paradigm change in psychoanalysis*. New York: Norton.

Stern, D. B. (1997). *Unformulated experience: From dissociation to imagination in psychoanalysis*. Hillsdale, NJ: Analytic Press.

Stern, D. B. (2010). *Partners in thought: Working with unformulated experience, dissociation, and enactment*. New York: Routledge.

Stern, D. N. (2004). *The present moment in psychotherapy and everyday life*. New York: Norton.

Trevarthen, C. (2001). Intrinsic motives for companionship in understanding: Their origin, development, and the significance for infant mental health. *Infant Mental Health Journal, 22*, 95–131.

Tronick, E. (2001). Emotional connections and dyadic consciousness in infant-mother and patient-therapist interactions: Commentary on paper by Frank M. Lachmann. *Psychoanalytic Dialogues, 11*, 187–194.

Tronick, E. (2003). "Of course all relationships are unique": How co-creative processes generate unique mother-infant and patient-therapist relationships and change other relationships. *Psychoanalytic Inquiry, 23*, 473–491.

Part II

Group analysis

Chapter 8

The Edge of Chaos

Enactment, disruption, and emergence in group psychotherapy

> To plunge into the unknown from what is known, but unbearable.
>
> —Bela Bartok (Demeny, 1971)

Introduction

In this chapter, I will introduce an approach to group therapy that is based on the idea that group psychotherapeutic process and change involves a constant movement into and through enactments that involve the group as a whole, the group analyst, and each group member. It is a truism in the group therapy field that a group is always interacting. This group interaction is the primary unique resource of group psychotherapy. It is out of this interaction that each group develops its particular group culture and the "group matrix" (Foulkes, 1975) from which change and growth emerge. As the group members engage with each other and bring in their whole personalities, enactments are unavoidable, and just like interaction, inevitable. In this chapter, I will examine the process of these enactments from the perspective of current relational theorizing that emphasizes the presence of multiple self-states in the group and the embeddedness of the group analyst within the group enactments. These enactments are constantly unfolding and involve the group as a whole and the group analyst in repetitive and unmentalized states. Therapeutic action, in part, involves the ongoing work on the part of the group analyst and group members in attempting to understand what is going on in the group. This is achieved by accessing alternative self-states that allow the therapist or group members to think about and try to understand what is happening and thus turn unmentalized (Fonagy et al., 2002), "un-understandable" (Pines, 1998), and painful interaction into psychological learning and development. This process often involves the group and the group analyst entering into difficult and sometimes painful passages of group process together. With the therapist's help in containing the painful and disowned affect, new experience and meaning can emerge for the group members from the unmentalized, unformulated, and rigid repetitive self-states that characterize the enactments.

The primary dynamic of change is conceptualized as a constant dialectical movement into and out of the "familiar chaos" (Stern, 1997) of the self-states engaged in the enactments and the more reflective and related self-states that enable working through. In order to describe this process and to outline the experience of the analyst's embeddedness, I will look to dynamic systems theory that offers a conceptualization of change and emergence that seems to capture the experience of these enactments both systemically and metaphorically and is beautifully captured by Stuart Kauffman's (1995) notion that "life exists at the edge of chaos," to hermeneutic psychoanalysis that emphasizes the emergence of meaning from dialogic interaction, and to relational psychoanalytic ideas of enactment, dissociation, and multiplicity.

The work of the group and enactment

As the group therapist, my task is primarily to create and maintain the safe, productive, and transformational space within which the group can do its work. I set the boundaries of the group and help and encourage the group members to work together to create a dynamic group that is itself the agent of change. Rather than therapy *in* the group, I am working toward a situation where there is therapy *by* the group (Foulkes, 1975).

It is not uncommon for the group to engage in what feels like chaotic, painful, or numbing interactions with each other and with me. Most often, these interactions are variations on the very damaging, deadening, and mystifying dynamics of the group members' lives and minds. When these internalized modes of experiencing themselves and others unfold, it is often as familiar, repetitive patterns in relationships that are experienced as unthought "things that happen." They leave the individuals with a dead and helpless feeling about themselves and the sense that this is "just the way things are." At times, there is tremendous pain and turbulence generated for the individual and the whole group by these ways of being. These interactions are versions of early trauma to the self that has taken place before there was sufficient language or cognitive ability to mentalize and thus construct a meaningful narrative, or later trauma that has been dissociated and has not been available for mental processing. This kind of damage to the mind and its relations to the world is not amenable to being talked about; it can only find expression via projective identification and enactment. My work is to help the group find what is meaningful and coherent in these chaotic interactions and to allow the emergence of what has until now been unformulated (Stern, 1997) and stuck in the realm of what cannot be thought and felt.

Rather than overcoming resistances or lifting repressions so that the unconscious can be made available, I see this work as the facilitating of a creative and emergent interactive group process wherein what was unformulated can take shape and find meaning. I help the group members work together such that the multiple and sometimes incompatible parts of themselves come to be enacted in the group. These enactments always involve the individual members themselves, the group as a whole, and the therapist. Everyone is involved.

Time and the emergence of meaning in group therapy

Group therapists almost universally talk about the focus on the "here-and-now" in group therapy (Ormont, 1992; Rutan & Stone, 2001; Yalom, 1975): Patients are encouraged to talk about their experience in the here-and-now. Often, focus on past events or on future hopes is questioned as an avoidance or flight from what is going on in the here-and-now (Ormont, 1992). My focus on the emergence of unformulated experience in group enactments takes a somewhat different view to the trajectory of time in group psychotherapy. The focus is on what is *happening* in the group and what will *emerge*. The distinctions between past, present, and future dissolve when the focus shifts to the finding of meaning in the what-is-about-to-emerge. Whether group members are talking about past experience or their feelings in the moment is less relevant. The point is that either way, they and the other members are, or soon will be, doing something with each other that may itself contain the pieces of unformulated experience that need to be allowed to emerge and take shape within the group. Hans Loewald (1980) used the phrase "near future" to capture the curious transference enactments wherein the past is continually lived as an about-to-be future. It seems useful to think of the life of the group as taking place in the transformational space that is the "near future," or as the French poet Yves Bonnefoy (1982) puts it, "the ever next."

The work of finding meaning rather than repetitive deadness is itself a reparative and restorative endeavor. The British group analyst Malcolm Pines (1998) has eloquently described how the group evokes the primary mother-infant emotional environment and can become a space and an object in and of itself that contains the qualities of mirroring, relatedness, and reparation. Group members respond to and internalize these qualities over time. My hope is that they not only find situations that promote the making of meaning out of their empty and unthought experience, but also that they will internalize and develop for themselves the reflective function and the ability to mentalize that emerge within the group (Fonagy et al., 2002). These capacities are initially embodied in my being, presence, and attitude in the group.

The hermeneutic circle and unformulated experience in group

From a hermeneutic and constructivist approach to group psychoanalysis, the unconscious is not regarded as a storehouse of complete and inert memories, objects, and experiences waiting to be unearthed and brought to consciousness via interpretation (Hoffman, 1998; Orange, 1995; Stern, 1997). Rather, the meaning of behavior emerges through the group interactions and dialogue. The hermeneutic contribution to psychoanalytic process builds on Gadamer's (1975, 1976) conception of the hermeneutic circle. Meaning is conceived as "an activity, an event" that "can only take place in interaction" (Stern, 1997, p. 212). Although originally applied to textual analysis, the relevance to group interaction is compelling. Meaning emerges as we test our assumed understanding in dialogue with an other. Our understanding shifts as our preconceptions have to be adjusted to account for what we do not yet understand or only partially understand. One way to think about the interaction of group psychoanalysis is a version of the hermeneutic circle wherein the members are trying to be understood and are trying to understand the others in the groups. Gadamer (1976) has emphasized that the act of trying to understand a text or an other is transformative in itself. There is an ongoing process of adjusting and readjusting perceptions and assumptions in order for a shared meaning to emerge.

This transformation of the self and creation of meaning is the very process that has broken down for the patients who come to group. Rather than being open to alternative perspectives about their own ways of being and an openness to know the other group members fully, we find that they are locked in a repetitive "familiar chaos." This is a phrase that Donnel Stern (1997) borrowed from Paul Valery. He describes a "state of mind cultivated and perpetuated in the service of the conservative intention to observe, think and feel only in the well worn channels – in the service, actually of the wish not to think" (p. 51). Such a state of mind feels familiar and therefore a comfort, and yet is chaotic in that experience and thoughts are yet to be developed or formulated. It is a state of mind that is dissociated in that there is a failure to construct or make sense of what is happening. Things just happen. Such a conceptualization is not far from Bion's (1962) concept of "-K" or "anti-thought." The as-yet unformulated experience is not accessed through interpretation, because there is nothing there yet to interpret. The unformulated experience can only be known if allowed to emerge in the group process, and to take shape and meaning in that emergence.

In group psychotherapy, there is a constant dialectical movement between enactments of the familiar chaos of the patient's lives and the search to find the meaning in these enactments. (In truth, the word *multilectic* would be more appropriate, given that *dialectic* implies a dialogic pattern between two poles – as in Hegel's thesis and anti-thesis – while in the group therapy situation we are looking at a situation where the multiple self-states of the group and its members intertwine in a multitude of enactments and reflective states at any given time). The leader is often involved unconsciously in the enactments along with the other group members, either in a dyadic manner or in terms of a group-as-a-whole enactment. The task of the leader and the group is to try to notice when these enactments are occurring – in everyday speech, "to figure out what's going on" – to describe the experience and then to try to make sense of it. The exercise of making and finding meaning in the enactments gives shape to what is unformulated as it is emerging and is transformative in itself.

Complexity and multiple self-states in group

This constant movement between the rigidity of dissociated repetitiveness and the freedom to think new thoughts and find meaning finds resonance in the application of complexity theory, or dynamic systems theory, to psychoanalysis (Galatzer-Levy, 2004; Ghent, 2002; Harris, 2005; Palombo, 1999) and group therapy (Rubenfeld, 2001). Outlined in an ever-expanding literature, (Gleick, 1987; Lewin, 1999; Waldrop, 1992), complexity theory offers a way of thinking about the clinical experience of group and individual psychoanalysis that goes beyond linear and binary explanations (Harris, 2005). The group may be viewed as a self-organizing eco-system that is subject to the processes of all biological systems; like all biological systems, any perturbation to the system will cause changes to the whole system. A group, like any open system, will settle into attractor states that offer relative stability. These attractor states can be shallow and therefore vulnerable to complete reconfiguration in response to perturbations or can be deep and far more resistant to disruption.

Rubenfeld (2001) points out that unlike earlier notions of General Systems Theory (Agazarian, 1989; Durkin, 1981; von Bertalanffy, 1966) that conceptualized a group, like all living systems as drawn toward equilibrium and homeostasis, complex systems – and a psychotherapy group is a superb living example – must maintain *dis*equilibrium and *in*stability in order to adapt to changes in the internal and external environment. Rather than seeing a group as always engaged in maintaining homeostasis, this view sees groups as always engaged in adapting to new and changing circumstances. In particular, perturbations to an open system cause destabilization and turbulence that then open up the opportunity for change.

In the group therapy situation, there are manifest perturbations to the system, such as the arrivals and departures of members, vacations, and the like. (There are also constantly more subtle and perhaps smaller perturbations such as the shifts in self-states within the group members from one moment to the next). As the vignette to be described below illustrates, such events can cause terrific personal and group turbulence, and powerful opportunities for change and growth. It is in the most turbulent times that vulnerable group members are more prone to rely on the more rigid and known patterns of their own "familiar chaos" as a first order adaptation. Familiar and protective self-states are called upon to manage the terrors of change. It is out of these self-states that enactments are born, as the whole group and the therapist may get pulled into a dissociated self-state that does not allow access to other more adaptable and flexible self-states that would allow for the formulation of the experience. As we will see below, a self-state that allows thought and mentalization can be a rare and precious commodity at a time of such turbulence.

Stuart Kauffman's (1995) concept that "life exists at the edge of chaos" highlights the ongoing tension in all living systems between rigidity and sameness, on the one hand, and disruptions, chaos, and change, on the other. This is what happens in group psychotherapy when there are perturbations to the system and old familiar ways of coping that involve the dissociation of more flexible self-states operate. From this perspective, this is what enactments involve: a cleaving to a familiar and worn pathway of being and not formulating experience (that is, dissociating) in the face of turbulence.

Both complexity theory and contemporary relational psychoanalysis offer us ways to focus on the fine-grained moments when there are shifts from one state to another, from dissociation and enactment to reflection and the creation of meaning. In the field of complexity and mathematics, there has been a shift from the prior held truth that there are three classes of behavior – fixed point, periodic, and chaotic – to the addition of a fourth class: an intermediate class between fixed and chaotic (Lewin, 1999). Lewin (1999) describes how these ideas were adapted to the world of cell life and then to eco-systems by Kauffman (1995) and others. It appears that all biological life is sweetly poised at the "edge of chaos" where "chaos and stability pull in opposite directions" (Lewin, 1999, p. 51). What is so compelling to psychoanalysts and group analysts is the idea that it is the intermediate area between order and chaos that offers maximal information processing, change, and creativity. This area is termed the "edge of chaos."

In systemic terms, the group and the individual members involved in trying to find their way through an enactment are poised in that fourth zone between the fixed and chaotic – within and between dissociation and the formulation of experience – and it is here that there is tremendous opportunity for powerful emotional experience and change. Such a moment can also be conceptualized as the "phase transition" (Lewin, 1999, p. 20), where the disruption has been sufficient to shift the system out of one attractor state and the system has yet to settle into the next one.

The phrase "the edge of chaos" also speaks eloquently to the phenomenology of these situations. As the vignette described below hopefully conveys, for the group members and the therapist, there is an exquisite alchemy of pain, disruption, and new insight, and experience when an enactment is allowed to emerge and is worked through.

From within the field of relational psychoanalysis, Philip Bromberg's (1998) image of "standing in the spaces" within and between different self-states also speaks to the phenomena of enactments in group psycho-therapy. I suggest that this resonates with the above idea of the fourth zone of experience that is between the fixed and the chaotic. The very task of interacting with each other and living out the group interactions, while simultaneously engaging with the task of figuring out what's going on, asks the group therapist and the group members to inhabit at least two self-states at once and the space between them: one that permits an immersion in the experience of the moment with the other members, and the other that seeks to mentalize, to find the meaning and shape of that experience. In other words of Bromberg's, how do we "stay the same while changing"? Bromberg (1998, 2006) has given us many compelling clinical examples that highlight the immense value of careful attention to the shifts in self-states in the patient and in himself in individual work. Similarly, the work of group therapy is conducted right "at the edge of chaos," that is, when there are shifts in the self-states of the group-as-a-whole, the members, and in the group analyst.

The group analyst and enactment

Often, when the group-as-a-whole is engaged in a blind and total way, the group analyst is unable to maintain his or her analyzing function and stay in the self-state that will offer insight or at least some connection to the task of the group to try to understand their experience. Unlike other approaches to group-as-a-whole phenomena and to group therapy, a rela-tional approach does not assume that the group analyst can stay outside of the enactment with the clarity that enables accurate and meaningful inter-pretations of the group process. Indeed, the idea that the group therapist is immune to group-as-a-whole processes and can maintain clarity of con-sciousness while the group members are swept away in the unconscious group process is seen from a relational perspective as both undesirable and actually impossible. Steven Mitchell (1993, 1997) has persuasively reconsidered the analyst's authority and knowledge as entirely mediated by the analyst's own experience and subjectivity. It is only by becoming lost in the total experience of the group – or as Donnel Stern (1997) puts it, the "grip of the field" even if that involves a temporary destruction of thought processes (Hinshelwood, 1994; Gordon, 1994) – that one can find and create meaning in the enactment. In situations such as this, the analyst has to work hard to help the group stay in touch with the task and to try to find one or some parts of some of the members who can begin the process of mentalizing and reflective function that will guide the group out of their temporary darkness. Experiences such as these are drenched in pain and struggle for the group members and the group analyst, but are the *sine qua non* of a group therapy experience that will be real and vital and will actually bring about change.

In order for this kind of process to emerge – to be "lived out," as Betty Joseph (1985) would say – the group therapist must be able to contain and hold the group while the enactment unfolds. Premature interpretation, the rush to know something before it has come to be, in the group – or in Betty Joseph's words, to turn the experience into analytic "material" – can impinge and constrict the group's potential to live through and find their own meaning and grounding in the experience that unfolds. The hermeneutic approach values the idea that there is no one correct meaning to the group's behavior, and I would always value the meaning that the group comes to from within their own struggle together over any interpretation I might be able to offer.

An enactment of disruption and emergence in a group session

As by now will be clear, my approach to group psychotherapy embraces the idea of disruption and turbulence. Far from being a problem to be overcome, disruptions to the group mindset and to the group itself are seen as opportunities for growth and for the shifting of self-states. What follows is part of a session of an ongoing group in which we will see the group's response to another disruption in a sequence of disruptions. The session will illustrate the dialectics of enactment: the rigid repetition of "familiar chaos" as a response to disruption and turbulence, on the one hand, and the emergence of new and invigorating meaning from within that enactment, on the other. Here is a group living at "the edge of chaos."

This is a weekly psychotherapy group that has been ongoing for ten years. There are six current members, two of whom have been in the group for the duration. The most recent member, Karen, joined approximately nine months ago, and both the membership and the feeling in the group in that time has been one of increasing solidity and stability.

Two months prior to this session, I moved office after eight years in the same office. This was a major disruption in the life and minds of the group.

There were various enactments of the loss of object constancy and going-on-being that this event called up in the group members. For instance, Victor forgot about the existence of Karen, and Gladys insisted that she would leave the group and that I was "a fucking bastard" for "dragging her around." As is often the case during disruptions such as the move, there really is a feeling of living on the edge of chaos. At one and the same time, there is a feeling of the reliving of all the past traumas and also of new and durable experience being made as the group goes-on-being and survives the storm.

The following session takes place four weeks after the move to the new office. All six members are present.

> It is in the group's culture to make all announcements at the beginning of the group session. Accordingly, I announce that there will be a new member coming to the group soon. There is a swirl of energy in the room, mostly centering around curiosity as to whether the new person will be a man or a woman. Karen (the most recent member) is upset and says "Oh no; I was just beginning to open up. I hope it's not someone with an eating disorder. Those eating disorder groups are so competitive and insane. I'm thinking of doing DBT. But I don't have to do it on Wednesday night [group night]." By way of background, Karen is in her mid-30s and has had years of treatment after a massively traumatic childhood. She has struggled for years with all the disorders of trauma and neglect: difficulties in self-regulation, self-injury, eating disorder, and on two occasions was hospitalized when suicidal. Karen had indeed only recently begun to open up and talk more intimately about herself in the group. When she is anxious, her speech and thought are disjointed and muddled as they are here. My thought is that her disjointed fragmented state is capturing the whole group's state of mind in response to the news of the new member.
>
> Gladys speaks up and says that she's thinking of leaving the group. Dorothy says that a new member makes her think of how long she has been in the group (she is one of the founder members) and that she still finds the group useful. She still learns a lot. Victor chimes in: "Me too." Victor and Henry review their respective progress in the group and talk for a few minutes in a disconnected way. Both Victor and Henry are prone to this kind of reverie in the group and can talk in a dissociated way when there is anxiety and turbulence brewing

in the room, as if to ward it off and to repair the fragmented group. Both come from families where anger and fear can suddenly erupt in parents or siblings with frightening intensity. While they are talking, Gladys's face darkens. I am aware of this, and anxiety wells up within me. I am aware of charging my batteries; this is going to be a long night. I ask the group, "What's going on?" Karen asks Gladys "Are you okay?"

Gladys turns to me slowly and malevolently: "I hate you. I was just getting over hating you for moving. I was going to leave the group, but then you moved and I couldn't leave because it would seem like I was leaving because of that and I'm busy with work and now this! Now I can't leave because it'll seem like it's because of the new person, not because of my own reasons. I'm just going to leave. I want to go off my meds. I'm sick of it. Isn't that meant to be how it goes: You get better and can cut down, but Dr. B says they are helping so why change. But I'm just going to leave."

I scan the room. Heads are down. The mood is grim.

I address the group: "How are people feeling toward Gladys?"

Victor leans toward her: "I feel supportive. I know what you're going through. You don't have to feel that way."

Henry picks up the thread, once again joining with Victor in the attempt to soothe the rage and fear in the room. He responds to Gladys's comments about her medications and launches into a long disconnected story, all too familiar to the group, about his trials and tribulations with his thyroid medication. It should be mentioned that Henry is an intellectually brilliant man, the son of scientists who seem to relate to people as if they were robots, with little sense of human functioning. He often feels other than human and can only relate in this very split-off, affectless manner. Since being in the group, he has begun to be and to feel more a member of the human race.

I encourage the group to find out what Henry feels at this moment, but it's not so easy to shift Henry from his groove. After a few failed attempts, I ask the group what is Henry feeling toward Gladys, that he doesn't know. There is unison. He doesn't want her to leave; they cry. Henry looks pleased. "Yes," he says, "Please don't leave." There is a small ripple of pleasure in the room. Henry has found a feeling. However, Gladys is still drenched in darkness and everyone knows it.

Gladys ignores the group and Henry. She focuses on me again: "I hate you. I was just getting comfortable with you again. I had been so angry and was just feeling okay with you, and now you're doing this again! She continues for a time in dark hatred. I ask her to say, if she can, what is it that I am doing to her. "You're just taking it away from me. I can't leave now. I hate you."

I try to reflect – "I've trapped you" – but she is not yet in a state that will permit ingress.

She continues. "I know what it is. You need more money. I know it, once you moved in here. The new office; you'll need new furniture. You gave us a chance to settle in and now this!"

I try again to reach her: "You feel annulled. If I move, I'm annulling you. If I raise fees, I'm annulling you. Like you said when we moved, I'm just dragging you around"

She has heard me, especially the reference to being dragged around, her own words, spoken when the group moved, that resonated with her feeling as a child, but she is still trapped in her familiar chaos. She has responded to the disruptive news of the new patient with a fall back into the repetitive rigid familiar chaos of traumatic neglect and annulment.

She continues: "I can't go on. I just can't do this. I need to leave. I'm not coming back. I'm going back to school in the evenings in September so I'll have to leave anyway. It's just too much. Up to now, everything I've done has been arranged around the group and my therapy schedule. I've organized my vacations around group and my individual sessions. Now you do this!"

The atmosphere in the room is vile, ugly, and hopeless. I am not doing too much better. I can feel the dark pull of Gladys's self-state. I see the rest of the group sucked into her darkness. I am distraught. We have been into and through these passages before with Gladys, and it is always slow and painful. It can take weeks until the group comes out the other side. I am deeply upset and experience a collapse within me into a complementary self-state. I become certain that I have made a grievous error inviting a new member in at this time. I am quickly on the slippery slope of self-denigration. It is all falling apart. How could I have made such an error? How can I possibly think I can run groups, let alone think of writing about and teaching group therapy? I convince myself that there is no alternative but to cancel the new group member. I think of all the repercussions of this: the conversation I will have to have with the patient and the referring clinician and so on. I am now locked in the enactment with Gladys and the group. I feel that I am a terrible persecutory and neglectful object who has no business running groups. In retrospect, in Heinrich Racker's (1968) terminology, I imagine that this was a complementary version of Gladys's mother's unmentalized dread that she was not up to the task of having and raising children. Similarly, in a concordant way, the group and myself are experiencing the unmentalized, dissociated piece of Gladys's upbringing. We are feeling bullied and tortured by her pain and rage, as she was by her mother. It is a victimized response that leads to an internal collapse that involves self-denigration, helplessness, and disgust.

In the moment of the group, I am, as Donnel Stern would say, "in the grip of the field." I cannot see or feel alternatives at that moment. The group is in the same grip. In such situations, I use the multiplicity of the group. I look to see if there is anyone in the group who can access a different self-state that can offer a way out of this grip and open the path to thinking.

So I ask the group what people are sitting with. Henry says that he's thinking that we shouldn't forget that the group could be of great benefit to the new member, too. There is the slightest perceptible shift in the feeling in the room. Henry, perhaps due to his affective disconnection or to his response to the previous moment where the group and I helped him express a deep and simple feeling toward Gladys, is not entirely stuck in the group self-state of horror and helplessness with and in response to Gladys. He is a little more able to stand in a space that allows him a perspective and allows him to think an empathic thought about the needs of the new member. He is able to feel that the new member is herself a subject, not just an object. In this moment, he is free of the enactment in a way that neither the group nor I can be. Such openings of thought and intersubjectivity in the midst of an enactment are enormously helpful. I am able then to function in a somewhat freer way myself. I notice that Dorothy is looking particularly pained, and I become sure that she is responding to Gladys. I ask her what she is feeling toward Gladys.

Dorothy says: "To be honest, and I hate saying this, but Gladys, the first part of what you said made me angry. And I hate saying this because I know that you are in a bad place. But I couldn't help but feel 'oh no, here we go again; now this bad place that Gladys is going into is going to fill up the whole group,' and I really can't stand it when you say that you are going to leave. It hurts me so much. In fact, what I feel, and I hate saying this, is that I think I feel what you say you feel when your sister does what she does to you. It's like it completely takes over and there's no room for anyone else. Then we all have to go along with it and we can't challenge you or even help you."

This is a major shift in the self-state of the group and for Dorothy personally. Dorothy has spent her life being cowed into submission by an officious academic family where the men were valued over her and where no expression of anger was ever tolerated, especially in the only girl. Now a senior administrative professional, she is often presented in her work life with situations that require assertion and confrontation, and she struggles mightily. This is why she keeps saying how much she hates saying what she is saying.

Gladys does not look at Dorothy while she talks. She looks away and seems to boil with rage. She turns to me again.

"Well it's your fault. I did nothing. You did it all. You moved! You are bringing new people into the group!" Hatred spills out of her, and I feel for Dorothy who is now being annulled by Gladys.

At this point, my feeling state has changed dramatically. I am not lost in the grip. Henry and Dorothy have helped us to stand in the spaces. We are still in the grip of the field created by this enactment, but we are also, in different ways, able to think about and mentalize the experience.

I tell Gladys that I think that she feels very vulnerable, and that she then feels she has only two options: to attack or to run away. I ask her, can she let herself be vulnerable here?

Dorothy says to Gladys: "But I'm not blaming you."

Gladys continues to act as if she's ignoring Dorothy and more hatred toward me comes out, and she insists that she is leaving the group.

Dorothy now erupts in tears of sadness and rage. She says, "That's it then. I'm never going to speak in group again. I express my feelings and you see what happens. You just attack."

Gladys responds to her. This is a sign that she is also able, ever so slightly, to step out of the traumatized overwhelming self-state. She says, "I'm just saying what I feel."

Karen says, "I also have to say I felt like oh no, here we go again. This is going to take us over for the next few groups. I also feel like I don't want to deal with a new person. Look Gladys, you are not going anywhere. I've seen you like this before. You're still here."

Henry, Victor, and Karen then talk for a while about how difficult group can be, but they emphasize the virtue in being able to express whatever feelings arise. The effect is a distancing from the heat of the moment, but it is not unwelcome, as it seems to have given Dorothy and Gladys a moment to think. This is an example of the group's self regulating capacity.

Dorothy says to Gladys with more softness in her voice, "Look Gladys, you really hurt me when you say those things."

Gladys, also with more openness says, "But it's not my fault, it's his [Grossmark's] fault."

Dorothy responds, "But it's no one's fault. That's not what I'm talking about. Not blame. I'm just saying that I felt angry. I didn't want to, but I just felt I needed to express it. No one is being blamed."

I amplify Dorothy's point, sensing that Gladys is now shifting to a self-state of openness and thought. I tell her that this seems to be just how it goes in her family. There is no room for vulnerability and need. It's always about someone being blamed.

Gladys cries. She shakes with anger. "I'm so fucking angry with my sister. You won't believe what's going on. She's pregnant again!"

This has the quality of a bombshell. The group has worked hard over the last year to help Gladys cope with the overwhelming disruption, envy, and isolation she has experienced following her sister's first pregnancy and the birth of her first child.

The group is gripped by this news and the self-state of the group is now utterly vibrant and engaged. Gladys tells a story of family dysfunction. Her sister isn't speaking to her parents and is angry with her. Everyone engages in the conversation that feels full of vitality, empathy, and sharing.

The group finds its way out of the enactment

How did this group release itself from the grip of this painful enactment? Or, in the terms of dynamic systems theory, what facilitated the phase transition out of the attractor state of the enactment. First, Henry introduced the subjectivity of the new member. Then Dorothy tried to express her emotional reaction to Gladys's assault and persevered in her attempt to have her own subjectivity acknowledged. When Dorothy implored Gladys to understand that she was really hurt by her and that no one is to blame, she was implicitly calling to the other potential self-states that Gladys can occupy. She was reaching out to the part of Gladys that can empathize with Dorothy and that can have what Fonagy and his colleagues would call "reflective function." Finally, Karen too was able to step back and in an empathic manner tell Gladys that she was not going anywhere. In that moment, Karen and Gladys were standing in a new dialectical space. Karen was saying, in effect: "You are in this awful place and I have been pulled into it with you, but you and I know there are other parts of you, other self-states which still exist even if you cannot reclaim them right now." All of these interactions are the building blocks of emotional meaning and mentalization that allow the group to make a new intersubjective and related experience out of an old repetitive enactment of familiar chaos and dissociation.

Group leadership, containment, and complexity

It is primarily by creating the space within which the group could live through this enactment that meaning and the potential for change emerged. There were many opportunities to intervene with interpretations about what was going on. From the get-go when Karen talked in her fragmented way, I could have commented that this was a reaction to the news of the new member. Certainly later many interpretations were possible when Gladys began her assault. Such attempts to turn these moments into group "material," I believe, would foreclose the enactment and deprive the group of the experience of living through these experiences together and to finding their own meaning and mutual help within the experience. The rush to interpret or give premature closure to such moments are often driven by the analyst's anxiety and can be understood as the analyst's need to dissociate (Reis, 2006). It is hard and disturbing for the analyst to be pulled into such dark places. My work is not to do the group's work for them or to know what is going on before they do; my work is to maintain the frame and contain the intolerable affect and thereby help them to do this work together. This involves allowing my immersion in Gladys's assault, to allow it ingress, to become temporarily stuck in the self-state of self denigration and collapse, and to be available with the other group members when an alternative self-state is evoked that will allow us to stand in a space both within the enactment and outside of it.

The group then is in the presence not only of an object that maintains the frame and is durable in the face of disruption and attack, but also an object that is affected and moved along with the group. Alvarez (1992) talks about an "animate object" that facilitates the growth of a human mind by joining with and responding to the needs of the child. She elaborates on Winnicott's (1971) idea of the use of an object that emphasizes the object's survival of the infant's attacks. She paints a picture of an object that facilitates the process of reparation following the envious and hateful attacks of the infant or patient. For Alvarez, the process of reparation is crucial to the development of the child's mind and central to the process of containment. What seems to relate most pertinently to my role in the group is the focus Alvarez (1992) places on the changes that the object of reparation undergoes: "A repaired object . . . is fundamentally different from an undamaged one" (p. 142). In the group, I believe that one part of me, one self-state, is available to be temporarily damaged and then restored, to be disturbed and then to recover, and to be changed in the process. This facility is the animate and alive version of containment that promotes reparation and the growth of mentalization. Similarly, Bollas (1987) suggests that the analyst must become disturbed by the patient when there is powerful disturbance and distress present.

This is a different conception of the role of the group leader. Such a group leader is effective by being engaged, moved, and changed along with the group. This leader operates within the group and yet is always maintaining the safety and boundary of the experience. This is a conception of leadership that seeks to integrate the idea of complexity in systems and is guided by the position of the relational analyst: mutually yet asymmetrically engaged in the process of emergence and change (Aron, 1996).

In terms of dynamic systems theory, the leader is no more able to stay out of the attractor state – the enactment – than the group. The influence that will perturb the system sufficiently to enable the transition out of the attractor state, is most potent when coming from within the group itself, as when this group finds its way to alternate and mentalizing self-states. The leader's role, then, can be conceptualized as the managing of the phase transition or the period of disequilibrium and instability and allowing for this to emerge from its own process. The leader's role is to live with the group at the edge of chaos.

Implications for technique and the group analyst's subjectivity

In terms of group analytic technique, there are a number of considerations that my approach suggests. In order for this work to be possible, it is of primary importance that the frame and boundaries of the group analytic situation be maintained as firmly as possible. Without the experience of a firm yet responsive frame around the group, the patients cannot enter into the kind of emotional territory and exploration described above. Further, without confidence in the frame and the group members' adherence to all the group agreements (Rutan & Stone, 2001), such as not socializing outside of the group and maintaining confidentiality, the group analyst cannot feel comfortable allowing the development of such enactments and will not be able to tolerate the emotional strain for him or herself.

The maintenance of the frame also involves an appreciation of the group analyst's role as leader of the group and the powerful group dynamics and transferences that leadership evokes (Bion, 1962; Klein et al., 1992; Turquet, 1974). The relational approach has, however, introduced a critical reconsideration of the role of the analyst and the analyst's neutrality (Aron, 1996; Hoffman, 1998; Mitchell, 1993, 1997). As mentioned above, it is no longer considered helpful or even possible for the group analyst to be perched above the dynamics of the group in such a way that objective interpretations of the group process are possible. Such a position asks that we also reconsider the role of disclosure of the group analyst's subjectivity during the group and in particular during enactments such as the one described here.

My guiding principle is to always act according to what will maintain the safety of the group environment such that enactments can unfold as deeply and revealingly as possible. Accordingly, it is important that the group analyst be both comfortable and mindful when bringing his or her own subjectivity into the group. I do so when the heat of the group is milder, which is to say, when there are multiple self-states available in the group such that, first, I can find my own subjectivity (not a given during powerful enactments), and second, that my subjectivity can be comprehended by the group members. For instance, on another occasion, Karen experienced Victor as bullying her. The group members were in agreement with Karen and talked about their feelings about Victor. I had not experienced Victor in this way and introduced this to the group for consideration.

When I introduce my subjectivity in this way, it is in the spirit of inquiry and curiosity, that my perception at this time is one of many possibilities. This, I feel, is important in that it not only values the members many points of view, but also models the open search for meaning and self-reflection that I hope will become a part of the group culture. On this occasion, I was also mindful that Victor can fall into the role of scapegoat, and that Karen can find injuries where there is the smallest slight. In this instance, the atmosphere in the group was one of curiosity and exploration, and my introducing my subjectivity was stirred into the mix of the discussion in what seemed to be a healthy manner and furthered the spirit of inquiry (Lichtenberg et al., 2002) and reflection prevalent at the time.

When the group enters the territory of powerful enactments where self-states become rigid and dissociation predominates as described in this chapter, I am much more focused on maintaining the safety of the enterprise. In a situation such as this, I suspect that revelation and discussion of my sense of fragmentation and despair would have created more terror and trauma in the group members and would have therefore closed down the unfolding of the enactment, rather than allowed it to continue. In situations such as this, the containment of the experience seems to be of the utmost importance. To have injected my own experience at this particular juncture would, I believe, have been an evacuation of the difficult emotions I felt I was being asked to contain. My evaluation was that there was little reflective function available in the group at this point and that all I could do was to hold on to the experience and neither preclude nor evacuate it. It is my ability to hold on under duress, to search for my own reflective self-states, that will be internalized by the group members over time.

In conclusion

I have illustrated an approach to the theory and practice of group psychoanalysis that utilizes the relational concepts of multiple self-states, the centrality of enactments, and the emergence of meaning and mentalization within them. A theory of healing in group psychoanalysis emerges that emphasizes the analyst's containment of enactments and the value of turbulence in group process. The dynamic systems theory concept that change and growth occur in the moments between order and chaos is applied to the group process, particularly to the moments where the group members stand in the spaces within and between alternative self-states while searching for a way through an enactment.

In the vignette, the group members were not only helpful to Gladys, but as I hope is clear, were becoming less reliant on dissociation themselves, while growing their own abilities for reflective functioning, mentalization, containment, and intersubjective relatedness.

References

Agazarian, Y. M. (1989). Group-as-a-whole system theory and practice. *Group*, *13*, 131–154.

Alvarez, A. (1992). *Live company: Psychoanalytic psychotherapy with autistic, borderline, deprived and abused children*. Hove: Brunner-Routledge.

Aron, L. (1996). *A meeting of minds: Mutuality in psychoanalysis*. Hillsdale, NJ: The Analytic Press.

Bion, W. R. (1962). *Learning from experience*. Northvale, NJ: Jason Aronson.

Bollas, C. (1987). *The shadow of the object: Psychoanalysis of the unthought known*. New York: Columbia University Press.

Bonnefoy, Y. (1982). *L'Arriere-pays*. Paris: Gallimard.

Bromberg, P. M. (1998). *Standing in the spaces: Essays on clinical process trauma and dissociation*. Hillsdale, NJ: The Analytic Press.

Bromberg, P. M. (2006). *Awakening the dreamer: Clinical journeys*. Mahwah, NJ: The Analytic Press.

Demeny, J. (Ed.). (1971). *Bela Bartok letters: Letter to Mme. Muller-Widmann, October 14, 1940*, pp. 284–285.

Durkin, H. E. (1981). The technical implications of general systems theory for group psychotherapy. In J. E. Durkin (Ed.), *Living groups: Group psychotherapy and general system theory* (pp. xx–xx). New York: Bruner-Mazel.

Fonagy, P., Gergely, G., Jurist, E., & Target, M. (2002). *Affect regulation, mentalization and the development of the self*. New York: Other Press.

Foulkes, S. H. (1975). *Group analytic psychotherapy: Method and principles*. London: Gordon & Breach.

Gadamer, H. G. (1975). *Truth and method*, G. Barden & J. Cumming (Trans. & Ed.). New York: Seabury Press. (Original pub. German, 1960.)

Gadamer, H. G. (1976). *Philosophical hermeneutics*, D. E. Linge (Ed.). Berkeley: University of California Press

Galatzer-Levy, R. M. (2004). Chaotic possibilities: Toward a new model of development. *International Journal of Psychoanalysis*, *85*, 419–442.

Ghent, E. (2002). Wish, need, drive: Motive in the light of dynamic systems theory and Edelman's selectionist theory. *Psychoanalytic Dialogues*, *12*, 763–808.

Gleick, J. (1987). *Chaos: Making a new science*. London: Penguin Books.

Gordon, J. (1994). Bion's post-"Experience in Groups" thinking on groups: A clinical example of -K. In V. L. Schermer & M. Pines (Eds.), *Ring of fire:*

Primitive affects and object relations in group psychotherapy (pp. 107–127). London: Routledge.

Harris, A. (2005). *Gender as soft assembly*. Hillsdale, NJ: The Analytic Press.

Hinshelwood, R. D. (1994). Attacks on reflective space: Containing primitive emotional states. In V. L. Schermer & M. Pines (Eds.), *Ring of fire: Primitive affects and object relations in group psychotherapy* (pp. 86–106). London: Routledge.

Hoffman, I. Z. (1998). *Ritual and spontaneity in psychoanalytic process: A dialectical-constructivist view*. Hillsdale, NJ: The Analytic Press.

Joseph, B. (1985). Transference: The total situation. In M. Feldman & E. B. Spillius (Eds.), *Psychic equilibrium and psychic change: Selected papers of Betty Joseph* (pp. 156–167). London: Routledge.

Kauffman, S. (1995). *At home in the universe*. New York: Oxford University Press.

Klein, R. H., Bernard, H. S., & Singer, D. L. (1992). *Handbook of contemporary group psychotherapy: Contributions from object relations, self psychology and social systems theories*. Madison, CT: International Universities Press.

Lewin, R. (1999). *Complexity: Life at the edge of chaos* (2nd ed.). Chicago: University of Chicago Press.

Lichtenberg, J. D., Lachmann, F. M., & Fosshage, J. L. (2002). *The spirit of inquiry: Communication in psychoanalysis*. Hillsdale, NJ: The Analytic Press.

Loewald, H. W. (1980). *Papers on psychoanalysis*. New Haven, CT: Yale University Press, pp. 43–52.

Mitchell, S. (1993). *Hope and dread in psychoanalysis*. New York: Basic Books.

Mitchell, S. (1997). *Influence and autonomy in psychoanalysis*. Hillsdale, NJ: The Analytic Press.

Orange, D. M. (1995). *Emotional understanding: Studies in psychoanalytic epistemology*. New York: Guilford Press.

Ormont, L. R. (1992). *The group therapy experience: From theory to practice*. New York: St. Martin's Press.

Palombo, S. R. (1999). *The emergent ego: Complexity and coevolution in the psychoanalytic process*. Madison, CT: International Universities Press.

Pines, M. (1998). Psychic development and the group analytic situation. In M. Pines, *Circular reflections: Selected papers on group analysis and psychoanalysis* (pp. 59–75). London: Jessica Kingsley Publishers.

Racker, H. (1968). *Transference and countertransference*. New York: International Universities Press.

Reis, B. (2006). Even better than the real thing. *Contemporary Psychoanalysis, 42*, 177–196.

Rubenfeld, S. (2001). Group therapy and complexity theory. *International Journal of Group Psychotherapy, 51*, 449–471.

Rutan, J. S., & Stone, W. N. (2001). *Psychodynamic group psychotherapy*. New York: Guilford Press.

Stern, D. B. (1997). *Unformulated experience: From dissociation to imagination in psychoanalysis*. Hillsdale, NJ: The Analytic Press.

Turquet, P. M. (1974). Leadership: The individual and the group. In G. S. Gibbard, J. J. Hartman, & R. D. Mann (Eds.), *Analysis of groups* (pp. 349–371). Washington, DC: Jossey-Bass Publishers.

von Bertalanffy, L. (1966). *General systems theory and psychiatry*. New York: Basic Books.

Waldrop, M. M. (1992). *Complexity: The emerging science at the edge of order and chaos*. New York: Simon and Schuster.

Winnicott, D. W. (1971). *Playing and reality*. London: Tavistock.

Yalom, I. D. (1975). *The theory and practice of group psychotherapy*. New York: Basic Books.

Chapter 9

Narrating the unsayable

Enactment and the creation of
meaning in group psychotherapy[1]

Introduction

In this chapter, I outline an approach to working with unformulated and
non-represented experience in group analysis. This approach highlights
the hermeneutic nature of group enactments and regressions and concep-
tualizes these enactments as narrations and representations of what has
yet to have shape and form. I will describe enactments in group treatment
of what has happened but is yet to be experienced and symbolized, and
also enactments of what has never happened, or of what was lacking: the
consequences of neglect. I will illustrate how allowing group enactments
to flow and find full expression can enhance the emergence of narrative
and meaning where hitherto there had been empty repetition, pain, and
absent-mindedness.

As a psychoanalyst and group leader, I am always focused on the idea
that treatment is by the group rather than by the leader. From this perspective, the group is always doing and creating: the group is always telling a story, sometimes consciously in words and often in a way that is
completely outside of awareness of the members. Narrative and meaning
emerges in what the group is doing, in interaction and in behaviors with
each other, in the eloquence of action. From this perspective, one is always
focused on what the group *is* doing, on what *is* emerging rather than on
what they are not doing or what is being resisted or avoided.

Groups, meaning-making, and the flow of enactive engagement

It is a truism to say that groups are always interacting. As they do so and
group members engage with each other, enactments are unavoidable, just

like group interaction. Enactments are constantly unfolding and involve group members, the group analyst, and the group-as-a-whole. There are constant oscillations between rigid, dissociated, and unmentalized states that often cause pain and turbulence for the group and analyst, and more reflective states where the group and the analyst have more space to think and to relate. It is in interaction and enactment that we find meaning evolving. Here I draw from contemporary psychoanalysts who have emphasized the hermeneutic aspect of treatment (Orange, 2010, 2011; D. B. Stern, 1997, 2010). The touchstone here is the philosophical work of Hans-Georg Gadamer (2004). Meaning does not exist such that it can be interpreted, but rather comes into being through enactment itself, through dialogue and intersubjective engagement; meaning is not regarded as a linguistic formulation, it is an event. This perspective shifts the nature of the therapeutic action of group and individual treatment. There is a move away from the idea that therapeutic action derives from the interpretation of meaning as a static truth that can be analyzed intellectually from the outside, as it were. From the hermeneutic perspective, the work of healing involves the creation of meaning in interaction and enactment. The emphasis here is on the engagement and the emergence of what has yet to be known, in interaction. Meaning is to be lived through together, to come into being.

As outlined in Chapter 2, I have called this mutual process the "flow of enactive engagement" (Grossmark, 2012b, 2015a), a kind of lived, shared free association or free-floating discussion as Foulkes (1948) described it. The patient and analyst, or group and group analyst, together surrender to the regressive process that emerges between them and can flow together into psychic and emotional territory that offers new and often surprising meaning. Rather than Freud's (1913) original metaphor regarding free association of a solitary subject reading off the images that pass by the train window, we now have a contemporary metaphor of an intersubjective and shared endeavor where both participants in an individual treatment sit *side by side* as they are taken by a process that they both constitute and are constituted by, into realms neither could have foreseen. In the group setting, understanding and meaning are thus emergent and are *lived* together in the flow of enactive engagement, rather than cognitively arrived at: a true Gadamerian conversation in which narrative is a relational event.

From this perspective, there is a subtle shift toward a different image of the power of group. Classically, group therapy has been regarded as a way to situate the patient in a regressive situation. The emphasis has been on the regressive pull of the group situation and group dynamics (e.g., Schermer & Pines, 1994). I believe that anyone who has experienced any kind of group, whether small or large, can attest to the evocation of more regressed phenomena. However, I would propose that this is not the *only* aspect of group process that is available for the group and its members. I would suggest that we can fruitfully think of regression as the evocation of different self-states (Aron & Bushra, 1998), perhaps more fragmented, less developed, more emotionally charged, and so on. I would foreground the primarily creative potential that these self-states offer. I am not here talking about artistic creative potential, although these self-states may also be the font of actual artistic or scientific creation. Rather, I am talking about the potential to create experience and meaning that had not been realized before. I am proposing that when a group is unobtrusively allowed to flow through enactments in a safe way, tremendous creative potential to make meaning where previously there was emptiness and dull repetition is freed up. Being a part of this creative and vitalizing enterprise is in and of itself a healing experience for many members even when they are not the specific object of the group's work.

From this perspective, the role of the group analyst is to create the conditions that foster and unobtrusively protect this flow into and through enactments (Grossmark, 2012a, 2012b). He or she is not regarded as being outside of the group process such that interpretations can be made from a perch that is unaffected by what is transpiring in the group. Because dissociated and unformulated experience emerges in enactment and in relatedness, it is assumed that the group analyst will unconsciously play a part in the unfolding narrative. It is paramount, therefore, that the analyst is available to utilize his or her subjectivity to amplify whatever process is emerging within and between the group or individual patient and analyst. The group analyst pays careful attention to whatever snags and chafings (D. B. Stern, 1997, 2010) arise in their own consciousness that alert them to the emergence of what they and the group have yet to know.

The unobtrusive relational analyst (Grossmark, 2012a) allows the emergence of whatever process emerges in the group (whether we conceive of this as the group-as-a-whole, the field of treatment, or the analytic third) and simultaneously stays out of the way of that process while knowing that he or she is embedded in it and participates consciously and unconsciously with engagement and authenticity. Such work is only possible when the individual, group members, and analyst feel entirely safe, and hence there is rigorous attention to the frame and boundaries of treatment.

Let me give an example. Here is a group working with a powerful enactment of trauma.

Susan, an Italian-American woman in her forties, told the group a story of terrible violation and abuse. She had been sexually abused by her male cousins during family summers at a country house. She had never told her parents or anyone at all until she told her individual therapist. She and her therapist had agreed that it would be helpful for her to come to group to work on her issues with dating and to try to talk for the first time with other people about the abuse. She told me about this in the consultation for group. I told her that she could take her time in group and to bring in the abuse only when she felt ready. For the first few group sessions she attended, she was a friendly and open presence, able to offer help to others. She talked mainly about her problems dating. However, the moment came, and after a few weeks, she told the group about the cousins and the violation and abuse. However, as she did so, she was visibly transformed and told of the abuse in a manner devoid of any affect. The atmosphere in the room became soured with the stench of abuse, perversion, and toxicity. Group members, many of whom had suffered terrible abuse themselves, reacted with violent intensity. Jenny was enraged that Susan's parents had not noticed or in any way protected Susan. Susan protested that her parents were exemplary. She had never wanted to upset them. Jenny's rage turned to fury, and she screamed that she wanted to burn the whole of Susan's family alive for what they had done. George, whose father had been incestuously involved with his younger sisters, wanted to know more details about the actual sexual abuse. Julian, who had been sexually abused by a neighbor as a child, said that he wanted to leave the room because he was feeling nauseous and accused George of being a pervert who was trying to get some kind of stimulation out of Susan's painful story. I myself was overwhelmed and feared for Susan's mental safety. I feared that she could not withstand this onslaught and would be re-traumatized. I told the group that these intense and terrifying emotions were of extreme importance, because we were entering into the actual experience of abuse and violation. In this group enactment, which continued over many sessions (interspersed with other self-states and forms of relatedness), the group came to live through what Susan had yet to experience. The affect – terror, pain, disgust, violence, perversion – that had been dissociated and unthinkable up to this point emerged within and between the group members. Furthermore, each of the other group members entered the fields of dissociated trauma that they had yet to fully experience: George's horror and contempt for his father, Julian's fear and revulsion, and Jenny's rage at her abusive parents all became activated in the group enactment. The group indeed felt for a while that it was "on fire" with intense affect and the combustion of previously dissociated and unformulated rage and terror. Gradually through many sessions, the group members were able to talk to each other with more reflective function and observe the dynamics of trauma and offer support for each other. For instance, George was able to say to Susan that he was sorry for his intrusive questions, but he understood that this was a terrible legacy of the incest in his own household. He had, in fact, been a compulsive snoop, at times even stalking women he had developed an interest in. He had never considered himself as anything but respectful of women. This perverse side of him was previously consigned to an alternate dissociated self-state, and regarded as "not me." Jenny asked Susan to understand her rage. Jenny connected to rage that she was previously unable to own. She listened carefully to the group's suggestions that she pushed people away with her burning rage at the whole world. Susan herself had never considered that she was angry with her parents. She gradually filled in a much fuller picture of a complex family system that seemed characterized by denial and dissociation. Most importantly, she began to experience affect as she talked about her family. She also began to reassess how it came to be that no relationship of hers ever lasted beyond a few weeks. She had always regarded this as simply bad luck.

A few sessions into the enactment presaged by Susan's revelations of abuse, I had a dream. I dreamed that Susan was on fire. I woke up with a clear thought in my mind. Susan, I thought, is a burn victim. And just like severe burn victims, she cannot be touched, because to touch her would cause even more unbearable pain. I thought of the many other possible psychoanalytic interpretations of the dream involving traumatic sexuality and violation of her body, her own aggression and its consuming quality, and so on. I felt all were useful in conceptualizing and understanding Susan. But I did feel, due to the clarity of my waking thought and the powerful visceral quality of the dream for me, that the idea of her as untouchable spoke most immediately to the group process and to all the other traumatized members of the group. They could not truly touch each other without unbearable pain. I shared this dream and my painful thoughts about it with the group. I told them that I felt that the members were trying to really contact each other, with all their trauma and pain.

The only way they could do so was in the fiery combustion of their traumas. The pain, aggression, and chaos were inevitable. The group itself was screaming a necessary scream. I do think that it was not only my thoughts about the dream as it related to what was happening that was helpful to the group, but also the felt experience of me as metabolizing and trying to make meaning out of the hellish pain that we were all gripped by, that helped them find the path through this enactment so that the group members themselves found their way to relate to each other from more than the one traumatized self-state.

The group had enacted all the parts of the violations and abuses suffered, and even perpetrated (in George's case), by the group members. They came to emotional life within the group sessions. The point here is that until the experience that has been dissociated and is yet to be narrated is actually lived through in an enactment, and is recognized and becomes graspable as lived experience in all its pain and sorrow, it cannot become "really real" and will remain as an invisible force (a dissociated self-state) impeding the patient's ability to live fully and meaningfully. Until such experiences as Susan's in the group, the events of her past had been "things that happened" but were not yet part of her self. They were empty of meaning for her. They were yet to be transformed via this lived and shared experience into "history," as opposed to "the past" (Bollas, 1995). All the members I have mentioned here were moved by the intensity of their own emotions during this period.

Trauma can be manifestly massive, such as that suffered by Susan and the other group members, or it can be subtle and almost everyday, such as the cumulative experiences of a child whose expressions of selfhood are met with controlling or shaming responses, or are disconfirmed by nonrecognition. These then become dissociated not-me self-states that can lead to many forms of symptomatology: We see, for example, the hardened concreteness of black/white thinking, disowned hostility, avoidance, and much more. The dissociated experiences become the story that cannot be told. Yet in group, the narrative unfolds as enactment and interaction. It is lived through and begins to become real and graspable. Susan had been unable to think beyond "bad luck" about her inability to make relationships work. Jenny had lived in quiet and lonely resentment, never considering that her own reservoir of rage might keep others from staying close to her.

Enactment in group psychotherapy

As this example attests, enactments often involve painful and abrasive interactions and experiences in the group. Rather than being seen as blockages or resistances to the harmonious working of the group, from this perspective, enactments are the very point of the exercise. The group with Susan may have felt for a while extremely difficult, even disorganizing, to the members and to me, but I do believe that the work that was done during this enactment was the very reason we were there. Indeed, the affective storm unleashed in the group after Susan's telling of her abuse opened up areas of emotion and experience that had not been available for these group members in this way before and offered a lived experience of containment and holding for these states and for the story to finally have form and hence meaning.

For me, the idea of enactment has helped me uncouple myself from the pejorative implication of the concept of "resistance." Hence rather than a resistance-based idea that would construe group process in terms of what is being avoided and not done, I would rather be curious as to what the group or group member *is* doing. I'd rather be curious and open to what is being created within the enactment, what story is being told, rather than divining what is not happening and what is being "resisted." As Thomas Ogden (2012) said from his neo-Bionian perspective:

> Transference activity . . . is a psychological act not of reliving infantile and childhood experience but, rather, the opposite of repetition of early experience – it is an act of experiencing for the first time (with the analyst and in relation to the analyst) an emotional event that occurred in infancy or childhood, but was impossible to experience at the time.
>
> (p. 41)

Treatment thus takes place through entering, living through, and finding some meaning and resolution through the enactments. Sometimes, these can feel benign, interesting, even quirky and entertaining; at other times, they can feel like entering an abyss of pain and torture. From a Bionian perspective, we might say that the group offers an apparatus for thinking these thoughts – a container – which is then internalized by the patients.

Non-represented experience in group analysis

Susan is a patient who had suffered massive trauma. What about patients who are more regressed: patients who are not so able to engage in a dialogic interaction and who barely recognize another self or subjectivity in themselves or in any others including the analyst (Director, 2009; Grossmark, 2012a, 2012b, 2013)? These are patients for whom there is little or no self or object constancy, for whom there are few alternatives to merger and the loss of self in human interaction. And what about states that are dominated by the absence of relatedness and contain earlier undeveloped, empty, and unspeakable parts of the self that can find no expression in language (Botella & Botella, 2004; Levine et al., 2013)? I would suggest that such areas of the self or self-states are much less likely to be reached by dialogic engagement. Such self-states are often chased underground, as it were, by a group treatment that puts a premium on relatedness, thought, and dialogic exploration. Such patients offer real dilemmas for the group therapist who is often interested in finding and working with feelings. For patients who harbor areas of blankness, emptiness, and deadness, feelings and emotions are often part of the false self adaptation to the world, their way of surviving and protecting themselves. Such patients may also be able to engage verbally, emotionally, and intelligently: They can appear to be engaged, when in fact the area or self-state that is frozen is an area that has no voice and no experience to express. They often appear uncomfortable in group, do not connect to others, dominate the group, or are themselves compelled to evacuate any potential thought or link to others by overly emotional talking or impingement on others. They are sometimes cold and haughty and often evidence symptoms that speak to an inner dysregulation of self, such as volatile affect and relationships, addictions and compulsions, and various kinds of sexual acting out and perversions. They are often lost in space and time and lack the regular coordinates that make life for most of us comprehensible and continuous. These patients are often confused in group and cannot tell what is wrong. They can only show! Often this "showing" involves what appear to be breaks in boundaries, lateness, non-engagement in the group, and actual missed sessions. There are many ways one can foreclose and misrecognize this showing. If any of these unconscious communications or silent screams from dissociated self-states are regarded as resistances or attacks on the frame of treatment, these self-states will be chased underground and become ossified and encrusted in even more unbearable shame. Here is an example.

Evan came late to group. I would rather not think about resistances to the task of the group or challenges to the frame of therapy. I'd rather let myself not know what is happening and try to see where the flow of the group enactment and my experience will take us, and anticipate the emergence of some as yet undefined meaning. Evan was a punctual and impeccably responsible person in his life. It turned out that he had been sleeping and had not woken up on time for the group. Evan had, however, been dreaming. I held in my mind the idea that one does not have to be physically present in the room to be in treatment, and asked about the dream. The dream was full of dread, loss, and being left. The group picked up on this profound theme in this man's life and gradually put together that they had experienced a painful absence when he had not shown up for group on time. One of the group members had talked with emotion about her dread that the late patient had forgotten about or even abandoned the group. I myself had harbored some similar worry. My take on this was that we were involved in an enactment. When the group expressed their feelings, what emerged was the articulation of a previously dissociated agony. The group played the part of the man as a child, dreading that he was emotionally abandoned and forgotten about, and the man himself inhabited the experience of being lost and forgotten as well as the role of the abandoning parent. When not interfered with, with too quick interpretations, the group can find themselves living out what had previously not been formulated. In its behavior, the group had told a story: his story, which he could not have told in words – and he was a man with considerable verbal gifts – because it was never formulated in his mind. He had never been attended to in such a way that his experience could be made real. The abandoned little boy was finally getting recognized and did not have to continue life as "not me." He did not have to live forever compelled to be obsessively thoughtful, punctual, reliable, and perfect to the point of psychosomatic anxiety symptoms.

This brief and very simplified example captures the idea that rather than seeing the patient or group as *not* doing something, as resisting, or as being lost, I would rather see what the patient or group is trying to create. I might see the patient as looking for, or even forcing, the therapist and group into some form of recognition of what the patient has yet to know about themselves. It is a silent scream from a dissociated self-state that the patient has had no access to. It is a scream that brings about the presence of an absence. *You cannot describe what has never happened.* Rather than trying to understand or interpret the situation, which might only lead to an intensification of the rigidity of the dissociated, not-thinking state, the therapist can unobtrusively welcome and engage in the flow of enactment with the other group members, and the meaning – as yet unformulated, unknown to the patient and group – will emerge in the interaction. It is in what happens and what is about to happen that the action of the group takes place. Only when something feels personally real for the group members and for the therapist, can it become truly known and have meaning. Certainly this applies to the first example of Susan's group: She and the group members I mentioned were silently screaming for recognition of their unformulated and unknown pain and trauma. Let me offer one last example of the emergence of the non-represented in a group.

Gregory was haughty and dismissive of the other group members. He seemed bored and irritated by almost everyone and everything. When first in the group, he briefly mentioned that he had been brought up in an abusive household where his father would become drunk and beat him and his mother. He related this with an absence of affect and a shrug that said, "Hey, what can you do?" He described his mother as an abused and limited person who had fallen into years of almost total silence and dull compliance with the father since his earliest years. He described her sitting in the kitchen talking to invisible people. She often seemed to be hallucinating. "But hey, what can you do? That's all in the past." He had, indeed, built quite a successful career for himself but struggled with friendships that often seemed to go wrong for reasons he could not describe. For the first two years in the group, interactions with him centered on repeated confrontations regarding his abrasive attitude to the group. At first aggressively abrasive when anyone suggested that he might do well to look at himself and his role in these interactions, he gradually seemed to trust that there may be something of value in the group, and he began to describe numerous situations in his life where he seemed to evoke discomfort and conflict, for instance, making members of his staff at work cry on more than one occasion and seeming to turn friends off. When telling the group about incidents at work that troubled, him he would, however, become lost in laborious details of who reported to whom, often mentioning many names and details of the organization that the group could barely follow. Typically someone in the group would ask for some clarification or would express confusion, and Gregory would become irritated and hostile, complaining that he was telling the group something important, if they could just listen to him! These interactions would often deteriorate into more abrasion and anger and typically end up with Gregory returning to his most frequent complaint: The group does not understand him, so what's the point of this anyway?

When trying to engage with others members of the group and with ongoing group process, Gregory would often seem to hold his head aloft and seemed to squint and peer at others in a manner that certainly looked like sneering. He literally seemed to look down his nose at others. Now this is not a group where the members hold back their feelings toward one another, and once again Gregory was on the receiving end of some pointed feedback as people told him how angry he made them and how hostile he seemed. He would say that he was surprised to hear this and insisted that he just wanted to engage. He seemed to make no connection with the group process and his problems with others at work and in relationships, even when the group would suggest that there probably was a pattern here worth looking at. One time, he described how he was completely mystified when a person he met at a social occasion had left the conversation with him in tears.

The pattern in the group continued, and he began to talk about leaving the group. Some group members appealed to him to stay; others said that they'd probably all be better off without him and his constant complaints. I told the group that I was very aware of the discomfort and misalignment between Gregory and the group and that I was most interested to stay with it and see what it was all about. I told them that I felt like we were all involved in a story but couldn't yet put words to this narrative. All we could do was to keep at it and try to be as honest and direct with each other as possible. The group and Gregory seemed calmed by this.

I certainly felt that his behavior could be well described as the projection of unmanageable anger and hatred into the group, such that he was constantly evoking anger in the group members, and the group members were identifying perfectly with the projections, creating a feedback loop of projective identification that had become the signature of his daily life. Such an idea would suggest that the clinical focus would be on the group and the therapist containing and metabolizing the anger until such time as he would be ready to "take back the projection" and integrate the anger into himself. Certainly, one could safely assume that he had good reason to be extraordinarily angry and scared of that and many other emotions, given the abuse and neglect of his upbringing. We could also focus on the enactment of an abusive connection. The group and myself would enact with him a version of the abusive and violently contaminated relationship with his father. There is no connection without pain and the loss of self, such that every interaction is laced with sadomasochism, and someone is always doing something onto someone else: There is simply never peace and easeful flow between people. Certainly, these ideas were floating in my mind when I said to the group that I felt we were part of a narrative that didn't have words yet, but I had that snagging or chafing feeling (D. B. Stern, 1997, 2010) inside that there was something more going on here, something outside of what could be thought or put into language. I think that if I offered these thoughts to Gregory and the group, there would have been general agreement that this made sense. I think Gregory himself would have felt understood by these comments and probably would have experienced some relief. But I wanted to listen to that unsettled feeling that I was sitting with and to keep paying attention to the group and my reactions. Something that was not formulated or represented was being enacted and lived in the group.

Gregory continued in the group, and over time, I began to notice that he often seemed distracted and continued to describe continual irritation with everyone in the group. In one group, he seemed particularly distracted. Another member asked what was up. He said that he was not able to follow the conversation and that he found himself totally confused. I finally had shifted my perspective enough to take his non-participation, his non-relatedness, seriously. That is, I felt his misattunement with the group and his constant criticism that he was not being understood was a big positive communication. It was not a communication about something that was NOT happening, but a vivid rendition of something that WAS happening between him and the group. He was unconsciously TELLING the group about his early years and his relationship with his mother. The group and he were living out a preverbal relationship that was characterized by the absence of attunement and organized thought. The question to ask in moments like this is not "What are you feeling?" nor is it to bridge in the way suggested by Ormont (2001) and others to ask other group members "What is Gregory feeling?" or even "What feelings is Gregory not able to have right now?" Such interventions focus on what is formulated, and as I mentioned, the articulation of feelings is often a way to not remain in a state of non-representation. So I just told the group that we needed some time with Gregory. The group fell silent and waited with me. Gregory seemed full of emotion and confusion. He started to talk in a way we had not experienced before. He said that he kept thinking about what Jimmy had said two weeks ago before he (Jimmy) went to visit his family out of state. Jimmy had said that he hates visiting his mother because she is so intrusive and insincere. Gregory seemed filled with emotion and could barely get the words out: "You don't know how lucky you are to have a mother: I don't have a mother." He seemed to be speaking from a very different self-state, a state that we had not yet encountered. Gone was the sneering and aggression, replaced by a self-state that seemed almost child-like in its clarity and naiveté. "I don't have a mother," he repeated. One group member gently said that we were aware of his mother's death some 15 years ago. Gregory continued to speak from this different self as every pair of eyes in the group was fixed upon him. His whole visage seemed transformed and open in a way that we had never before witnessed. "I don't have a mother"; "I want my mom"; "I want to know my mom." These words seemed to be spoken out of time, from a timeless childhood place from deep inside him. He wept uncontrollably and repeated the last invocation: "I want to know my mother."

Needless to say, this was a transformative moment for Gregory, for the group, and for my sense of him. His very simple plea – to know his mom – is not simple at all. If we cannot know and have access in a coherent way to our mother's mind, we cannot know and have good contact with ourselves. We are left with an absence, a void that has no words. In Andre Green's (1999) language, we are left with an area of an inner blank psychosis, of an internalized dead mother. Gregory's plea is not about the loss of his mother when she died; it is about the loss endured from his earliest moments of life, when there was a nothing where there should have been a something: a related, enlivened, and enlivening other. What Gregory had was an internalized blankness that suffused all of his functioning. He was continually out of sync with others and for the most part quite lost in human interactions. The internalized sadomasochistic relationship with the father became materialized in a self-state that afforded him protection, safety, and some sense of continuity as he engaged with other humans, all of whom threatened him. He "did unto others before they did unto him" as a way to stay vigilant and protect his extraordinarily vulnerable, empty, and unformed self that only existed in a non-represented self-state. This vulnerable self only emerged in this complex flow of enactment of misattunement and non-recognition in the group. This is the self that would have been lost if I had urged the group to articulate feelings prematurely, if I had perceived Gregory as resisting or attacking the group, or if I had promoted greater object relatedness via bridging (Ormont, 2001). In fact, he was showing the group an absence of relatedness that was yet to be known or to have any mental shape. And that showing emerged *in the group* as Gregory participated in the only way he could.

I think it is crucial in working in this area of non-represented and unformulated states to respect the group's capacity to create meaning together with the therapist and to be unobtrusive to this process, to not intervene and try to make something happen or to interpret too quickly. The unobtrusive relational group analyst is deeply engaged, open, and encouraging with the group and creates and protects the space within which enactments like this can unfold over time. This requires the group analyst to hold, contain, and metabolize many painful and complex feelings and states, and trust that the necessary narrative will unfold in the group.

The groups I have described in this chapter narrated what had been unsayable and unknowable for Susan, Gregory, and Evan. They created meaning where there had been absence, connection where there had been emptiness, and self where there had been only pain.

Note

1 A version of this chapter originally appeared as: Grossmark, R. (2017). Narrating the unsayable: Enactment, repair and creative multiplicity in group psychotherapy. *International Journal of Group Psychotherapy, 67*, 27–46.

References

Aron, L., & Bushra, A. (1998). Mutual regression: Altered states in the psychoanalytic situation. *Journal of the American Psychoanalytic Association, 46*, 389–412.

Bollas, C. (1995). *Cracking up*. London: Routledge.

Botella, S., & Botella, C. (2004). *The work of psychic figurability: Mental states without representation*. London: Routledge.

Director, L. (2009). The enlivening object. *Contemporary Psychoanalysis, 45*, 120–141.

Foulkes, S. H. (1948). *Introduction to group-analytic psychotherapy: Studies in the social integration of individuals and groups*. London: Maresfield Library.

Freud, S. (1913). Further recommendations on the technique of psychoanalysis: On beginning the treatment. In J. Strachey (Ed. & Trans.), *The standard edition of the complete psychological works of Sigmund Freud* (Vol. 12, pp. 121–144). London: Hogarth Press.

Gadamer, H. G. (2004). *Truth and method* (2nd rev. ed.). New York: Continuum.

Green, A. (1999). *The work of the negative.* London: Free Association Books.

Grossmark, R. (2012a). The unobtrusive relational analyst. *Psychoanalytic Dialogues, 22,* 629–646.

Grossmark, R. (2012b). The flow of enactive engagement. *Contemporary Psychoanalysis, 48,* 287–300.

Grossmark, R. (2013). The register of psychoanalytic companioning. Paper presented at *Colloquium of the Relational Track of the Postdoctoral Program in Psychoanalysis,* New York University, New York.

Grossmark, R. (2015a). Repairing the irreparable: The flow of enactive engagement in group psychotherapy. In R. Grossmark & F. Wright (Eds.), *The one and the many: Relational approaches to group psychotherapy* (pp. 75–90). London: Routledge.

Levine, H., Reed, G. S., & Scarfone, D. (Eds.). (2013). *Unrepresented states and the construction of meaning: Clinical and theoretical contributions.* London: Karnac Books.

Ogden, T. H. (2012). *Creative readings: Essays on seminal analytic works.* London: Routledge.

Orange, D. M. (2010). *Thinking for clinicians: Philosophical resources for contemporary psychoanalysis and the humanistic psychotherapies.* New York: Routledge.

Orange, D. M. (2011). *The suffering stranger: Hermeneutics for everyday clinical practice.* New York: Routledge.

Ormont, L. (2001). The craft of bridging. In L. Blanco Furgeri (Ed.), *The technique of group treatment: The collected papers of Louis R. Ormont* (pp. 263–277). Madison, CT: Psychosocial Press.

Schermer, V. L., & Pines, M. (1994). *Ring of fire: Primitive affects and object relations in group psychotherapy.* London: Routledge.

Stern, D. B. (1997). *Unformulated experience: From dissociation to imagination in psychoanalysis.* Hillsdale, NJ: The Analytic Press.

Stern, D. B. (2010). *Partners in thought: Working with unformulated experience, dissociation and enactment.* New York: Routledge.

Chapter 10

The unobtrusive relational group analyst and enactive co-narration[1]

Introduction

In this chapter, I turn my attention to group work with patients and states that are not amenable to dialogic engagement. I outline an application of the ideas articulated in the foregoing chapters – the unobtrusive relational analyst, the flow of enactive engagement, psychoanalytic companioning, and the eloquence of action – to psychoanalytic work with groups and foreground the concept of enactive co-narration described in Chapter 7.

Each group develops its own unique idiom and character, and the group analyst can be unobtrusive to its development and expression. The analyst unobtrusively companions the group in the flow of enactive engagement and in the emergent narratives of trauma and regression that emerge. The emphasis is on companioning the group as it flows into altered and transformative states. The group analyst is not regarded as outside of the group process and able to interpret from a domain of neutrality, from a "view from nowhere" (Nagel, 1989). He or she conducts the group from within and constructs and is constructed by the group process even as he or she occupies the distinct role of leader or conductor. Treatment is by the group. The members work with each other and companion each other into and out of enactments and regressed worlds of trauma and neglect. Words are present, but it is understood that, just as Balint (1968) so presciently observed, much of this work is outside of the domain of language and must remain so. This sentiment reverberates with the words of E. James Anthony (1983), when describing his experience of group work with S. H. Foulkes, the founder of group analysis. He wrote: "Perhaps the most valuable lesson I received from Foulkes was on the value of unobtrusiveness on the part of the therapist and on the limits of explicitness" (p. 30).

The flow of enactive engagement and enactive co-narration

The unobtrusive group analyst companions the group as areas of diffusion, confusion, and damage arise between group members and in the group-as-a-whole. These are manifestations of non-represented experience (Levine et al., 2013) and unformulated potential experience (Stern, 1997, 2010) that have yet to have form. This is the realm "where thoughts arrive as actions" (Bollas, 2011, p. 239). These are not experiences or memories that are "tellable" or relatable. They emerge as enactments in the field of the group between members and between members and the leader. Enactments show rather than tell, and there is a continuous enacted dimension (Katz, 2014) to the group process. The group analyst can be unobtrusive to this emergence but is deeply engaged and knows that he or she can only know a small portion of what is actually emerging. It is in the shared companioning of the group analyst and the group members in these hitherto inchoate aspects of self that coherence emerges and mind, mentalization, and self-other relatedness take root.

When the "flow of enactive engagement" (Grossmark, 2012b, 2015) of the group members with each other and the group analyst is allowed to unobtrusively unfold, the work of the narrative becomes manifest. The group will spontaneously tell many stories (Grossmark, 2017). These are not only told in words, but also in the shapes and narratives that emerge as the group process and interaction unfolds. This is enactive co-narration. The field of the group will come to capture and express the unconscious and yet-to-be-formulated potential experiences of this unique group with these unique members. Furthermore, the field of the group captures unconscious, non-represented trauma and dynamics from prior generations and historical ghosts of all participants (Davoine & Gaudillierre, 2004; Harris et al., 2016a, 2016b). The flow of enactive engagement in group is an interactive, engaged, and multi-personal version of the Freudian idea of free association, much like Foulkes's (1964, 1975) adaptation of free association to group analysis that he called "free-floating discussion." However, unlike Foulkes's "free floating discussion," the flow of enactive engagement involves the analyst as embedded in the enactment and foregrounds the enactive dimension, the embodied incarnation of trauma, and states of primal psychic functioning and regression.

Such flows of mutual enactment can capture and tell a narrative of past trauma of the patient's life (or his or her forebears) that has been dissociated and never formulated, or as Aron and Atlas (2015) have outlined, can tell a story of the future as new dimensions of relatedness emerge. And as Neri (2008) and other neo-Bioninan field theorists describe, such enactive co-narration can describe unconscious and yet-to-be-known aspects of the group itself. The key is that the analyst flows with the group into areas that have yet to find psychological shape and form in the group members' or the analyst's minds. The group analyst fully utilizes his or her "negative capability" (Bion, 1971). The companioning of the group in these emergent experiences evokes a field that is itself transformative. Elaborating on Bollas's (1987) transformative object, the whole intersubjective matrix of the group may be viewed as a crucible of transformation within which the members come alive and represent their yet-to-be-known selves and stories via enactive co-narration. The following example will illustrate how a narrative of the past is told, not in words, but becomes incarnated in mutual enactive co-narration in the group. The narrative of the future is in the process of being built as the group members together live through transformations of what had been isolated fragments or beta elements (Bion, 1962) into shared and companioned experiences.

An enactment of family trauma

Greta, an unmarried white woman in her mid-forties, has been attending this ongoing group for two years. She initially came to group for help with persistent depression and a growing feeling of despair that she would never find a life partner or advance professionally. She had been a lively presence in the group and was much liked by the other group members, but frequently fell into evacuative states, where it appeared that her only mode of managing internal anxiety and arousal was to speak in a pressured manner, often asking the same question of another group member over and over again. When she would fall into this mode, the group would become impatient with her, and she often found herself on the receiving end of both anger and desperation from other group members. I too would experience extreme agitation when she would go into this mode. They would appeal to her to slow down and to take a breath. Generally, she would fall into sullen disappointment and withdrawal on such occasions and would return the next week with some degree of insight. For instance, she might return the following week, apologize for her behavior, and say that she has realized that she lost touch with her feelings and made the others uncomfortable. Typically, the feeling that would have eluded her was anger or fear. On this occasion, she came to group and described a situation at work. Her manager was bullying her and was openly favoring a colleague of Greta's, and together the boss and the colleague had made fun of her. Greta had begun to realize that she was, once again, going to be passed over for a possible promotion. Both the manager and the colleague were substantially younger than Greta. Greta relayed the story with a mix of fury and disdain for her manager and her colleague, but also conveyed a sense of resignation. She said that there was nothing that she could do: "The dye is already cast . . . you know how it is." Some group members joined with her acceptance and resignation and agreed that it was too dangerous to swim against the current; one had better keep one's head down and live to fight another day. One of these was Doris, who had grown up with an abusive mother. Seeming to have frequently entered delusional states, her mother would single her out for slaps, punches, and verbal assault, while always idealizing the other children. Doris had left home as soon as she was able and had grimly worked her way through college and into corporate culture where she steadfastly climbed the ladder of promotions. She was now a senior manager in a large corporation and had no personal life at all. She dressed in muted colors and had a grey colorless pallor. She always spoke slowly and rationally, often with great insight. She was always unruffled by the storm systems that might break out in the group. Other group members were outraged with Greta and her work situation. They expressed anger with the manager and the colleague, but most predominantly with Greta herself for "taking it." Peter, who had grown up watching his mother bullied and beaten by his alcoholic father, was furious with Greta: "How could you let this happen? You have to stand up for yourself." He became agitated, and Greta herself complained that she actually felt bullied by Peter as he assaulted her with his frustration. Anthony, who grew up bullied and traumatized by his older siblings, took a more conciliatory tone with Greta but also agreed that she had to stand up for herself. The tension in the room heightened. It was as if the group was dividing itself into two gangs who were readying themselves for an all-out confrontation: the rational-appeasers versus the stand-up-for-yourself-and-fight proponents. As these two groups became increasingly angry with each other, Greta herself slipped more quietly into the background. She tried to get a word in, to clarify this point or that, but to no avail: The energy was firmly located in the stand-off between the two sub-groups, and the atmosphere was becoming very heated, even some-what threatening. Peter brought up past confrontations with Doris, and each became accusatory about the other. Finally, Greta turned to me with a "can you believe this?" look. I asked her to speak her thoughts. She said to me and to the group that she couldn't quite tell how she felt, but she was certainly aware that everyone was fighting and that she felt like she had become invisible.

I was aware that Greta had become quiet, but I did not fear for her. I did feel that even if she did not "stand up for herself" right now in the group, she was able to survive. I found the aggression intense, but not unsafe. This is a sense that I recognize. It is as if the group is displaying a narrative that has yet to have meaning. It is a zone where the emotions are real, but at the same time cannot be taken as literal. On one level, one can say that in this long-term group where all the members have known each other for some years, there is sufficient safety and holding such that they can enter into areas of real pain and aggression and know that everyone will survive and come back to work together regardless of the degree of contention and abrasion. From another perspective, I have come to regard these altered transitional group states as transformative and revelatory. They are real and not real at the same time. A story, or a number of stories, are being enactively co-narrated between and among the group members. I can be unobtrusive and allow the enactive co-narration to unfold. My work is to hold the environment, to be sure that it is safe and to respect this flow of enactive engagement, and to not obtrude with interpretations or questions as to how a member is feeling and so on. I wait for the point of contact with me, and this came when Greta turned to me with her questioning look.

So I asked her to say more and said to the group that I was not sure how to understand this tension and aggression but that some very power-ful emotions and interactions were underway. In saying this, I hoped to endorse and support the group members in whatever they might be feeling, and also to offer the holding that comes with the idea that there is meaning here, even if we cannot connect to it yet.

Doris took the lead and asked Greta what she meant when she said that she had become invisible. Greta said that when she was a child, her broth-ers and parents would fight. Things would become unbearably terrify-ing for her. There would be violence between the father and the brothers and often pushes and shoves would escalate to violent fights. Knowing that Doris had abundant knowledge of family violence, I asked Doris to stay with Greta. Doris said that she understood how invisibility was the only solution when the environment was so dangerous. The others now joined in the conversation, and the stand-up-for-yourself sub-group and the rational-appeaser sub-group began to talk to each other and to understand each other.[2] This is a sure sign of the maturing of the group process and opening of deeper levels of communication. The group session ended, and I reassured the group that although this was a hard session, it felt as if we were a part of a number of stories that were being told in the group. Anthony replied, "No kidding!"

Over the next few weeks, among other group dynamics and other members' work, the group returned a number of times to the zone of this enactment. The feelings and sub-groups would re-emerge and the conversation pick up as if time had stood still. As time progressed, there was more and more room for perspective and thought. The group and the sub-groups were not as vulnerable to becoming completely immersed in the experience. All agreed with me when I suggested that the group became Greta's family for a while. Doris helped Greta with the idea that when the men in the family engaged in their violent and aggression-fueled dynamic, she would become invisible. Doris ruefully related this to the "equation" of her own life where she has subordinated herself fully to the demands of work. The group talked with her at length about the degree to which she has erased any passion and vitality from her own life. During this discussion, Doris sighed and threw her head backwards. In doing so, her hair fell away from her forehead, revealing a completely new aspect to her face. Anthony spontaneously commented on how he had never seen her look like that before, and other group members joined in saying that yes, Doris is indeed a beautiful woman. They had never quite seen her so. She is always so covered up. Moments like this are signals of a group process and transformation. The unobtrusive relational analyst allows this process to continue unimpeded, at times embellishing the ongoing dynamic. In fact, I did chime in at this point and said that I too had felt the grey clouds part when Doris made that gesture.

All agreed that Anthony and Peter had come to be Greta's brothers and father in the group. Anthony and Peter agreed that they had lost track of Greta when they were so forceful in their views about her standing up for herself. Greta related the issue of invisibility and safety to her work situation and connected to how scared she actually felt at work, even though her manager and colleague were so much younger than her and she mainly felt contempt toward them. Peter talked about how much he had dreamed of being able to save his mother from the violent attacks of his father and with great pain connected to how enraged he had been with her, his mother, for not standing up for herself. He related this with great anguish and sorrow. He began to see how he repeatedly positioned himself as savior in his relationships with women. None of these relationships endured. Anthony related the urgency he felt toward Greta's passivity to his own fear of his own passivity and vulnerability, both in his own work environment and in his relationships with women where he would most commonly find himself avoiding any semblance of his own needs or fragility. And for him, too, no relationship had endured.

To return to Greta: She was moved, energized, and at times confused by all these events and seemed to cycle from a receptive mode where she could take a perspective and think about the group dynamic and how it replayed her childhood, to a return to the pressured, evacuative mode that we were all so familiar with. All the members agreed that they had become Greta's family for a while, repeating the very dynamic of danger, acrimony, and splitting that she had survived by becoming invisible. I suggested that we should also think about how her pressured mode was also a part of that dynamic. Greta agreed, saying that she actually feels safer when she talks incessantly even if she knows she can lose people when she does that. Anthony related to this and said that it was probably a way of keeping her numb and disconnected. Greta agreed and talked about how she has always felt that she and Anthony have a special bond, both having been bullied as youngsters. Peter, still immersed in the anguish in relation to his mother, said that he was realizing that the emotion he felt when Greta would become pressured and insistent was fear. This surprised him and the group, but together they talked at length and figured out that when his mother succumbed to the father's abuse, he felt utterly abandoned by both parents. He had always dealt with that fear by the fantasy that he could protect and save his mother. Peter cried deeply as he spoke about the layers of complicated emotions he was in touch with.

Living an experience together

When discussing the development of the child's self and what we would now call subjectivity, Winnicott (1945) emphasizes that the mother and young infant come into meaningful relation with each other when "the mother and the child *live an experience together*," and this experience promotes the "first tie the infant makes with an external object" (p. 152). This is the crucible in which relatedness and the comprehension of external reality grows. When the mother and baby are harmoniously in synchrony, there is a moment of illusion – "a bit of experience which the infant can take as *either* his hallucination *or* a thing belonging to external reality" (p. 152). The mother does not challenge the illusion, but unobtrusively lives *within* the illusion with the baby. The baby finds his or her way to reality and relatedness through living in the illusory world *with* the mother, and the mother "enriches" the illusion rather than dispelling it.

Likewise, the unobtrusive relational group analyst follows the group as it enters this transitional area that is both real and hallucinatory. The idea is, as Winnicott suggests, to not "challenge the illusion" but to "unobtrusively live within the illusion" with the group. In this way, the group and its members find their way to "reality and relatedness through living the illusory world" together. Like the mother, the group analyst "enriches" the illusion rather than dispelling it. For instance, I chimed in when the group responded to Doris's transformative moment when she threw her head back and the hair fell away from her forehead.

The group is always enacting and narrating. I did not view Greta's pressured speech or the enactment of emotional trauma and erasure as issues to be dealt with via interpretation or any attempt to promote a higher level of relatedness. Rather, I regard these as enactments that call from non-recognized and non-represented self-states for recognition and companioning so as to make them real (Grossmark, 2016). I include here behaviors and occurrences that are often regarded as resistances or treatment-destructive acting out. For instance, I have described how I understood a patient who missed sessions as conveying the devastation of abandonment (Grossmark, 2015), an experience that had no form in his mind and therefore could not be told in words. It was via the enactive co-narration and incarnation in the group enactment that the experience began to have a form and therefore could be approached as an emotional reality.

Hence I do not seek to interrupt this narrative emergence while it is flowing and arising. The therapeutic action derives from the group members living through this experience together, rather than reaching a precipitous "understanding" of what is going on. For this reason, I wait to engage until the group signals to me that they need contact, as when Greta looked to me and expressed her need for my felt presence. Likewise, I hold onto many thoughts I have about the group dynamics that are unfolding, preferring to respect the group's ability to titrate its own levels of stimulation and connectedness. For instance, I understood that not only was the group enacting the story of Greta's family, but there was also an embodiment of Greta's internal worlds. One could regard the adversarial sub-groups as manifestations of the warring parts of her own mind, her internal object world where passions and aggression (embodied by Peter and Anthony) were at war with her self-protective, traumatized self (Doris). I hold these thoughts and formulations in my own mind and understand that the therapeutic action derives more from my containing and metabolizing these thoughts rather than interpreting them to the group at this time.

While it would not be incorrect to understand this group process according to the unfolding transferences, such as Peter reacting to Greta as if she were his mother, I tend to feel that such understanding can flatten out the rich, multi-layered process that was unfolding. A transference interpretation emanates from the logic of projection (Bollas, 2009), whereas I am seeking to allow the emergence of the "logic of enactment" and the enactive co-narration where many stories come to be *lived through* at once. In the logic of enactment, the whole group, rather than just two members, were involved in this narration or incarnation of Greta's family.

Furthermore, as Aron and Atlas (2015) suggest, enactments can dissolve the linear trajectory of time. In this enactment with Greta, the group not only incarnated the dynamics and trauma of her early years, but also contained the presence of the psychic healing which, one hopes, presage her future health. Greta had not repressed the trauma of her upbringing. She could, and indeed had, told the story of her violent and terrifying family on many occasions in the group. It was not out of awareness. However, as her erasing and invisiblizing herself attests, she had dissociated and removed herself from the emotional and intrapsychic dimension of the trauma while it was happening and in any further telling of the events. She was condemned to endlessly repeat rather than to truly remember the experience (Freud, 1914). One of the hallmarks of families where there is so much abuse and violence is the absence of containment, the inner mental processes that foster the making of experience and thinking itself (Bion, 1962). Rather, such families are characterized by a proliferation of evacuation of emotion, conflict, and of the mind itself. Hence no one can think, and everyone reacts with intensity. Such environments are always emotionally and often physically dangerous. Greta was continually showing this aspect of her own mind and that of her family with her signature pressured talking that never seemed to contain meaning itself and would typically evoke anger and less contained feelings in the group. All along, she had been showing the group – telling, if you like – the story of the absence of containment. And this telling involved all the members of the group, including me. Recall that I too would feel so very agitated when she would go into evacuative mode. This is the logic of group enactment, the work of enactive co-narration.

The healing grows, I suggest, not from interpretations from a knowing group analyst or from the orchestration of greater relatedness between group members (Ormont, 1992, 2001), but from the group members living through this experience together. As Balint (1968) says, much of these experiences "cannot, need not, and perhaps must not, be expressed in words" (p. 174). It is the work of the unobtrusive relational group analyst to allow the flow of enactive engagement and to companion the group in this living through together. There is consilience between Winnicott's work on the development of the infant's subjectivity and "unit status," the subsequent work of developmental psychology (Trevarthen, 2001), the current emphasis on implicit relational knowing (Boston Change Process Study Group, 2007, 2010; Lyons-Ruth, 1998), and the recent psychoanalytic emphasis on being-with (Eshel, 2013; Reis, 2009, 2010, 2016). All would suggest that it is the group members' being-with each other and living this experience together that fosters the growth of the inner structures of mind – in Bion's language, the apparatus for thinking and containing. This is the foundation of self-continuity, relatedness, mentalization, and reflective function, all of which Greta began to grow in this work with the group. It is these qualities that provide the foundation for a healthier processing of the trauma that had persisted in a dissociated self-state and hindered her development at work and in relationships. Of course, this is group analysis, so everything that is said about Greta also applies to all the other group members as well.

I would also point out that this enactment did not only transcend time and place in that it embodied the past, the present, and the future simultaneously. Furthermore, it embodied both the positive and the negative aspects of the trauma. In other words, it contained the incarnation of what *had* happened as well as the embodied presence of what *had not* happened: a mother and family's containment. Many patients can describe in words at least some of what did happen, even if traumatic and damaging. Patients can rarely tell what did not happen. This is the work of the negative (Green, 1999) and the presence of the absence, of states that have no form due to the absence of recognition, companioning, and attunement that would have made them whole and coherent experiences (Levine et al., 2013). It is in enactment and the work of the narrative that such non-represented and non-cognized states and absences come to have shape and form and can be experienced. Hence Greta and the group enacted both the absence of containment and the growth of the presence of containment. It is via the continuous living through of these states in group as one or another member struggles with their issues that psychoanalytic healing and the growth of mind and emotional capacity develops.

Conclusion

I have spelled out how an unobtrusive relational group analyst can allow the flow of enactive engagement and enactive co-narration such that group members can companion each other and live experiences together so that containment, mind, and relatedness can grow in and between group members. The group process is healing in and of itself, and the group analyst is unobtrusive yet deeply engaged in this process.

Notes

1 A version of this chapter originally appeared as: Grossmark, R. (2018). The unobtrusive relational group analyst and the work of the narrative. *Psychoanalytic Inquiry, 38*. Reprinted by permission of Taylor & Francis, LLC.
2 I lean here on the work of Agazarian (2006), who developed a comprehensive approach to the understanding and utilization of sub-groups in group treatment.

References

Agazarian, Y. (2006). *Systems-centered practice: Selected papers on group psychotherapy*. London: Karnac Books.
Anthony, E. J. (1983). The group-analytic circle and its ambient network. In M. Pines (Ed.), *The evolution of group analysis* (pp. 29–53). London: Routledge and Kegan Paul.
Aron, L., & Atlas, G. (2015). Generative enactment: Memories from the future. *Psychoanalytic Dialogues, 25*, 309–324.
Balint, M. (1968). *The basic fault*. London: Tavistock.

Bion, W. R. D. (1962). *Learning from experience.* London: Tavistock.

Bion, W. R. D. (1971). *Attention and interpretation.* London: Tavistock.

Bollas, C. (1987). The transformational object. In C. Bollas, *The shadow of the object: Psychoanalysis of the unthought known* (pp. 13–29). London: Free Association Books.

Bollas, C. (2009). Free association. In C. Bollas, *The evocative object world* (pp. 5–46). London: Routledge.

Bollas, C. (2011). Character and interformality. In C. Bollas, *The Christopher Bollas reader* (pp. 238–248). London: Routledge.

Boston Change Process Study Group. (2007). The foundational level of psychoanalytic meaning: Implicit process in relation to conflict, defense and the dynamic unconscious. *International Journal of Psychoanalysis, 88,* 843–860.

Boston Change Process Study Group. (2010). *Change in psychotherapy: A unifying paradigm.* New York: Norton & Co.

Davoine, F., & Gaudilliere, J. (2004). *History beyond trauma.* New York: Other Press.

Eshel, O. (2013). Patient-analyst with-ness: On analytic "presencing," passion and compassion in states of breakdown, despair and deadness. *Psychoanalytic Quarterly, 82,* 925–963.

Foulkes, S. H. (1964). *Therapeutic group analysis.* London: Karnac Books.

Foulkes, S. H. (1975). *Group analytic psychotherapy: Method and principles.* London: Karnac Books.

Freud, S. (1914). Remembering, repeating and working-through. In J. Strachey (Ed. & Trans.), *The standard edition of the complete psychological works of Sigmund Freud* (Vol. 12, pp. 145–155). London: Hogarth Press.

Green, A. (1999). *The work of the negative.* London: Free Association Books.

Grossmark, R. (2012b). The flow of enactive engagement. *Contemporary Psychoanalysis, 48,* 287–300.

Grossmark, R. (2015). Repairing the irreparable: The flow of enactive engagement in group psychotherapy. In R. Grossmark & F. Wright (Eds.), *The one and the many: Relational approaches to group psychotherapy* (pp. 75–90). London: Routledge.

Grossmark, R. (2016). Psychoanalytic companioning. *Psychoanalytic Dialogues, 26,* 698–712.

Grossmark, R. (2017). Narrating the unsayable: Enactment, repair and creative multiplicity in group psychotherapy. *International Journal of Group Psychotherapy, 67,* 27–46.

Harris, A., Kalb, M., & Klebanoff, S. (Eds.). (2016a). *Ghosts in the consulting room: Echoes of trauma in psychoanalysis.* London: Routledge.

Harris, A., Kalb, M., & Klebanoff, S. (Eds.). (2016b). *Demons in the consulting room: Echoes of genocide, slavery and extreme trauma in psychoanalytic practice.* London: Routledge.

Katz, G. (2104). *The play within the play: The enacted dimension of psychoanalytic process.* London: Routledge.

Levine, H., Reed, G. S., & Scarfone, D. (Eds.). (2013). *Unrepresented states and the construction of meaning: Clinical and theoretical contributions*. London: Karnac Books.

Lyons-Ruth, K. (1998). Implicit relational knowing: Its role in development and psychoanalytic treatment. *Infant Mental Health Journal, 19*, 282–289.

Nagel, T. (1989). *The view from nowhere*. London: Oxford University Press.

Neri, C. (2008). *Group*. London: Jessica Kingsley Press.

Ormont, L. (1992). Orchestrating a group. In L. Ormont, *The group therapy experience: From theory to practice* (pp. 83–98). New York: St. Martin's Press.

Ormont, L. (2001). The craft of bridging. In L. Blanco Furgeri (Ed.), *The technique of group treatment: The collected papers of Louis R. Ormont* (pp. 263–277). Madison, CT: Psychosocial Press.

Reis, B. (2009). We: Commentary on papers by Trevarthen, Ammaniti & Trentini, and Gallese. *Psychoanalytic Dialogues, 19*, 565–579.

Reis, B. (2010). Performative and enactive features of psychoanalytic witnessing: The transference as the scene of address. *International Journal of Psychoanalysis, 90*, 1359–1372.

Reis, B. (2016). Monsters, dreams and madness: Commentary on "The arms of the chimeras." *International Journal of Psychoanalysis, 97*, 479–488.

Stern, D. B. (1997). *Unformulated experience: From dissociation to imagination in psychoanalysis*. Hillsdale, NJ: The Analytic Press.

Stern, D. B. (2010). *Partners in thought: Working with unformulated experience, dissociation and enactment*. New York: Routledge.

Trevarthen, C. (2001). Intrinsic motives for companionship in understanding: Their origin, development, and the significance for infant mental health. *Infant Mental Health Journal, 22*, 95–131.

Winnicott, D. W. (1945). Primitive emotional development. In D. W. Winnicott, *Through pediatrics to psycho-analysis* (pp. 145–156). New York: Basic Books.

Index